Discover Magazine's Vital Signs

Discover Magazine's Vital Signs

True Tales of Medical Mysteries, Obscure Diseases, and Life-Saving Diagnoses

By Dr. Robert A. Norman

Introduction by Corey S. Powell

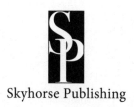

Skyhorse Publishing

Skyhorse Publishing books may be purchased in bulk at special discounts for sales promotion, corporate gifts, fund-raising, or educational purposes. Special editions can also be created to specifications. For details, contact the Special Sales Department, Skyhorse Publishing, 307 West 36th Street, 11th Floor, New York, NY 10018 or info@skyhorsepublishing.com.

Skyhorse® and Skyhorse Publishing® are registered trademarks of Skyhorse Publishing, Inc.®, a Delaware corporation.

Visit our website at www.skyhorsepublishing.com.

10 9 8 7 6 5 4 3 2 1

Library of Congress Cataloging-in-Publication Data

Norman, Robert A., 1955-
  Discover magazine's vital signs : true tales of medical mysteries, obscure diseases, and life-saving diagnoses/by Dr. Robert A. Norman.
    pages cm
  Includes bibliographical references.
  ISBN 978-1-62636-173-7 (alk. paper)
  1. Rare diseases—Miscellanea. 2. Diagnosis, Differential. 3. Medicine—Miscellanea. I. Discover (Chicago, Ill.) II. Title. III. Title: Vital signs.
  RC48.8.R68 2013
  616.07'5—dc23
                          2013024615

Printed in the United States of America

Many thanks to Corey Powell, Eric Powell, Steve George, Sarah Richardson, and all the editors and assistants at *Discover* I have worked with over the last fifteen years. Great appreciation goes out to Bill Wolfsthal, Wesley Jacques, Emily Houlihan, and all the staff at Skyhorse Publishing. Rita Rosenkranz, my super agent, helped me every step along the way to bring the book to fruition. Thanks to Tony Dajer for taking the time to read the book and provide comments. A special thanks to all the contributing writers who witnessed the birth of each of their stories and took the time to craft this fine collection. Much love to my family, friends, patients, and to all those that help fuel my creative energy and learning.

Note: The cases described in *Vital Signs* are true stories, but the authors have changed some details about the patients to protect their privacy.

TABLE OF CONTENTS

INTRODUCTION

By Corey S. Powell, editor at large and former editor in chief, *Discover* Magazine

For the patient, every trip to the doctor comes with a large dose of anxiety and intrigue. There is a fervent desire that whatever symptom prompted the visit has a perfectly benign cause—or, if it is a routine checkup, to find out that there is no cause in action at all. There is an always-present fear buzzing around in the back of the head that there might be something wrong. And then, still deeper down, the urge to know: If there really is a serious medical problem, what is it, what causes it, and what can be done?

One of the revelations of this anthology, a collection of the best "Vital Signs" columns that have run in *Discover* Magazine, is that doctors experience that mix of anxiety and intrigue too. The desired end result is also the same, of course: diagnosis, treatment, and—if possible—cure. But the path there is littered with obstacles, both personal and scientific. Patients are not always clear in describing their symptoms. Sometimes they lie, omit information, or fixate on extraneous or even imaginary details. Even accurate reporting can lead to an ambiguous diagnosis, and even a definitive diagnosis can lead to wrenching decisions about the best treatment.

Another revelation here is that these forty case studies are just plain great reads. Anxiety and intrigue are not just inevitable aspects of the doctor-patient interaction; they are also the essential elements of a mystery tale. So yes, each of the chapters in this anthology is a medical mystery, but they are also much more than that. They are character studies that examine the whole range of ways that people live and, in a few cases, how they die. They are meditations on the complementary processes of logic and intuition. They are pointillist-precise paintings of the ways that modern science seeks to control the biological processes that were once considered acts of fate.

And as you will soon see for yourself, these stories answer the question that many of us have wondered when looking at a doctor's illegible scrawl on a prescription pad: "Geez, can these people even write?" Yes, they can, and with remarkable insight and lyricism. No wonder, then, that "Vital Signs" was consistently the most popular section in *Discover*. It is the only column that has run the entire sixteen years that I've been with the magazine. It was the first column adapted to podcast and now the first column to inspire its own ebook.

Inevitably, you will bring some personal experiences along with you as you read these intensely human, personal episodes. I certainly did. The first things I recalled were two major health problems of mine that had concrete explanations. When I was eighteen, my shoulder erupted with a bumpy red rash that then continued in a line up my neck and onto the right side of my face. My physician took one glance and said, "Oh yeah, you've got shingles." I got it at an unusually early age, in a slightly unconventional location, but the diagnosis was straightforward. (The treatment, at the time, was to sit and wait it out. Fortunately, medical research has advanced at least a little since then.) Likewise when I was thirty and noticed a strange flickering in the left-hand periphery of the vision in my right eye: detached retina. A retinal cryopexy put things right, with only minimal damage to my sight.

But even in my mostly healthy life I have run into less clear-cut cases. That scary, recurring twinge of pain on the left side of my chest? Not heart disease, according to my EKG. Stress, maybe, or muscle strain from tossing my young daughters into the air too enthusiastically. Those odd red spots on my chest and arms? *Pityriasis rosea* perhaps, cause not entirely clear, treatment subjective—but at any rate, likely to go away after a few weeks. (It did.) And the peculiar dots, squiggles, and temporary subtle flutters that I occasionally notice in my vision? My retina specialist smiled reassuringly. "Those are nonspecific visual anomalies," he said. "Lots of people get them, they're not diagnosable, and as long as they are transient, they are not serious."

Many different symptoms appear on the upcoming pages. Some of them will be familiar to you personally; all of them will in some way echo experiences you have heard about from friends, relatives, colleagues, or the inevitable medical-themed TV shows. You'll meet people who visit the doctor or show up in the hospital complaining of dizziness, fainting, paralysis, seizures, hazy vision, weight loss, ringing in the ears. You'll encounter a child who grows inattentive, a woman who develops inexplicable lesions on her face and scalp, and a man whose irritable personality escalates into something more troublesome. And you will run into those vague lumps and sore spots that can mean nothing, or everything.

The range of diagnoses that unravel from those symptoms is equally expansive, reflecting the incredible complexity of the human biological machine and the near-endless number of ways it can malfunction. As you would expect, many of the major maladies make an appearance here: diabetes, heart disease, multiple sclerosis, pneumonia, cancer. So do common forms of self-damage, such as the abuse of alcohol and recreational drugs.

Then there are the truly confounding cases that a doctor sometimes encounters. How can you tell when a hypochondriac is really sick? How can you keep a sufficiently open mind to be ready for the truly freakish cases, such as a serious illness caused by . . . an oak leaf? But even the most well-known disorders take on unfamiliar form when they are seen as individual experiences, not as the kind of generic descriptions you find on Wikipedia or WebMD.

The path to diagnosis and treatment captured in this anthology similarly bears little resemblance to the kinds of neat checklists lists that so many of us now hastily consult before visiting a physician's office. (Perhaps we should call ourselves "impatients"?) The authors of these "Vital Signs" columns bravely expose their inner thought processes. They write candidly about missed clues, communication problems, administrative obstacles, overlapping interpretations of symptoms, the difficulties of processing information that may be incomplete or downright misleading. The doctors featured here are heroic in their intent, but they are not heroes in the classical sense. They are human beings—smart, dedicated, empathetic, but human all the same—doing their best to apply the lessons of two thousand years of medical knowledge.

By the time you finish this anthology, you will have absorbed a lot of that knowledge yourself, perhaps without even noticing. Even more subtly, you will have also completed a thorough course in ethics. A fruitful relationship between doctor and patient demands clear communication, trust, dedication, and compassion. Those same qualities are important in any meaningful life relationship, but rarely is their value so starkly laid out as it is in these stories.

In the end, the fourteen doctors who share their experiences here act both as experts in, and as witnesses to, the extremes of human behavior. Along the way they have picked up marvelous tidbits of wisdom. This whole volume abounds with memorable quotes. Insights into the medical mindset: "Neurology is what you do while you are waiting for the film to be developed." Insights into humanity's capacity for self-destruction: "He died from a combination of two of the oldest and most insidious killers of all: ignorance and avarice." Tidbits of hospital lore: "It's always the ones you don't worry about that you have to worry about."

And perhaps my favorite line in the whole book, for the deceptively simple way it sums up both the optimism and the lingering limitations of modern medicine: "It would be good to always be so lucky."

Corey S. Powell
Brooklyn, NY

CHAPTER

1

ATTACKED FROM WITHIN

By Robert A. Norman

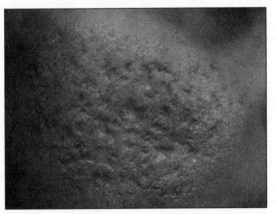

Photo 1-1

A 28-year-old woman sat on the examining table, pointing at patches on the sides of her face and scalp where it looked as if miniature grenades had exploded, leaving crevices.

"Can you get rid of them?" she asked.

"How long have those been there?"

"A couple of years. But now they're getting worse."

In addition to the lesions, I noticed a red, raised rash that spread across her cheeks, over the bridge of her nose, and around her eyes. I looked over her chart for medications and allergies. None were listed.

"So you don't take any prescription or other medications?"

"Nope. I just take a whole bunch of aspirin, or whatever I can afford, because my bones ache."

"Are you stiff when you first get up in the morning? Do your joints swell? How long does it last?"

These questions would narrow the diagnostic possibilities, but a skin biopsy and blood tests would also be essential.

"I'm going to need to take a small piece of skin to help make a diagnosis and get you better. I'll numb it up first," I said.

After removing a bit of tissue about the size of a pencil eraser from one of the lesions, I ordered a full blood count. I also ordered tests of kidney function, blood clotting, and liver function, along with an ESR (erythrocyte sedimentation rate—a marker of nonspecific inflammation), a CRP (C-reactive protein—another inflammation marker), and an ANA (antinuclear antibody) test. I suspected the patient was suffering from systemic lupus erythematosus, a widespread attack by her immune system on her own body. Experience told me that her symptoms would most likely add up to lupus, but I deeply hoped I was wrong.

"I'm going to give you a cream to put on your face to help clear it up and a pill you can take to cut down on your pain," I said.

As the test results rolled in over the next two weeks, the diagnostic picture became clearer. Although the result for C-reactive protein was normal, the ANA result came back positive. These antinuclear antibodies can turn up in patients on some prescription drugs, but when the result shows up in people not taking any of those drugs, it can be a sign of the immunologic problems of lupus. Still, I needed other results to make sure, and the biopsy offered one more clue. White blood cells along the junction of the dermis and the skin's more superficial layer, called the epidermis, are another sign of immune activation.

When viruses or bacteria attack the body, immune cells known as B cells normally respond by producing antibodies that bind to the invaders and mark them for destruction. In patients with lupus, the ability to distinguish one's own molecules from foreign molecules is disrupted, and the B cells produce antibodies that attack healthy cells and vital organs, especially the brain and the kidneys. Other immune cells, called T lymphocytes and macrophages, can also join the misguided attack on the self.

The symptoms of lupus are so varied that the disease can often go undetected for years. Common signs are arthritis, facial rash, and hair loss. Other manifestations include kidney damage, lung inflammation, and paralysis. Because lupus can disturb so many body processes, it often mimics diseases like scleroderma, multiple sclerosis, and rheumatoid arthritis.

Before a case can be classified as lupus, the American College of Rheumatology requires that the patient show at least 4 of 11 symptoms since the onset of the disease. My patient met that standard. She had the "butterfly" mark on her face, eroded red patches of skin in other areas, pain in the joints, and a positive ANA test. Like about 90 percent of all lupus patients, she was female and had developed the disease during her childbearing years.

Unfortunately, treatment options for lupus are still very limited. Cortisone and antimalarial drugs can combat inflammation by impeding immune-cell responses, and chemotherapy drugs like methotrexate and cyclophosphamide can curb the number of attacking white blood cells. Most recently, two cancer-related drugs have been used for treating lupus: mycophenolate mofetil, a drug that interferes with the metabolism of white blood cells; and rituximab, an antibody that kills B cells. But these medications all have side effects—cortisone thins the bones, mycophenolate mofetil can cause anemia, and methotrexate can irritate the liver—so the treatments require some sort of monitoring.

To suppress the immunologic flare-ups on her skin, I gave the patient topical corticosteroids as well as steroids injected into the lesions. I also sent her to a rheumatologist who put her on oral steroids and discussed other treatments. Over the next several months, we talked about the many problems she struggled with.

"I don't like this on my face," she said, pointing to the red rash. The butterfly rash, also known as the "red wolf" mark, is a classic feature of lupus. (In medieval times, contact with wolves was believed to cause rashes; lupus means "wolf" in Latin.) She shook her head in irritation. "People ask me everything from 'What did you get on your face?' to 'What the heck happened to you?' Now I'm losing my hair, and I'm growing hair where I don't want to. I wish I could take it and plant it in my scalp."

I recommended an excellent beautician and aesthetician. A good haircut and style would do wonders for her patchy alopecia; hair swatches or even full wigs can also help women with this condition. Special makeup, similar to what burn victims use, can minimize the appearance of scars.

"What else is happening?" I asked.

"Some days I can't eat because I'm sick to my stomach," she said. "People keep asking what's wrong with me. Then when I went on the steroids, I gained weight. And I get restless, can't fall asleep, and get all worn-out looking. I know I need the medicines, but sometimes I don't even want to look in the mirror."

Long-term use of immunosuppressive drugs can lead to a host of problems. While acne and changes in fat distribution are among the most visible adverse reactions, the list of potential side effects is long and devastatingly diverse: sun sensitivity, small sores in the mucosal lining of the mouth and nose, abdominal pain, diabetes, irritability, hypertension, cataracts, sterility, anemia, and other blood disorders. In some cases, high-dose corticosteroid therapy can also cause deterioration of the hip and knee joints. But the alternatives are worse. Patients who go without immunosuppressive treatment can face life-threatening kidney inflammation.

"Some days it feels as if it's my fault," my patient said. "I get to feeling real down."

I offered her what I could. Over time, she suffered less joint pain and her complexion improved. Perhaps most important were our talks about trying to cope with lupus. I confessed to her that I have always struggled with the lack of safe and effective medications for my patients with this cruel and chronic disease. I can only hope the future will bring better treatments.

Robert A. Norman is a dermatologist in Tampa, Florida, and the author of The Woman Who Lost Her Skin and Other Dermatological Tales.

CHAPTER

2

WHY IS GRANDPA FALLING?

By Tony Dajer

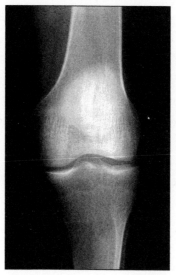

Photo 2-1

"Grandpa fell on knee. Two days before. Pain," the young woman said. Her wizened grandfather dozed on a stretcher. "How are you, sir?" I inquired softly.

In loud Cantonese, the granddaughter repeated the question. She smiled apologetically. "No hear good."

His eyes fluttered open. When I palmed his right knee, he winced. The joint was swollen, the kneecap scuffed, but he didn't complain when I bent his knee. With the help of an interpreter, I learned that he had tripped on his way to the bathroom two days before.

"No dizziness? No passing out? Didn't hit his head?" I asked. A yes to any of these questions would suggest more serious heart or neurological problems.

"No," the granddaughter replied. "Only tripped."

"He feels okay now?"

"Okay," she echoed.

The rest of his physical exam, except for weakness on his right side due to a previous stroke, was pretty darn good for an 85-year-old man.

His nurse appeared with the IV kit and blood tubes. "Admission labs?" she asked briskly.

"What makes you think he needs to come in?" I asked confidently.

"Grandpa fell," the nurse pointed out.

"It's his knee. Let's give him a Percocet. If the X-ray's negative, then he'll be good to go. We need the bed. And no Motrin, okay? He's already on Plavix and Persantine."

The latter two are potent anticlotting agents, and anti-inflammatory drugs like Motrin have a nasty way of making older stomachs bleed.

In the wild, animals past their prime face predictable perils: old hippos starve when their teeth wear out, and arthritic giraffes are felled by lions. For our bipedal species, the most dangerous environmental menace is gravity. Every year in the United States, one-third of people over 65 fall, risking not only a hip fracture but also a blow that can cause potentially deadly bleeding inside the skull. Compounding the risk for the elderly is the growing use of anticoagulants, which limit clot formation. Although these drugs help reduce the risk of strokes and heart attacks, they can turn a minor head contusion into a life-threatening gusher.

The patient's X-rays came back negative, as predicted. Hurrying into his cubicle, I announced, "Everything's okay—he can go home."

But the patient's visiting nurse had arrived to take over for the daughter. "So when will he go upstairs?" she asked.

"No, he doesn't need admission," I said.

Her brow furrowed. "You know, he has been falling a lot," she said carefully. "The family is worried."

My perkiness evaporated. A patient who frequently falls must be hospitalized to prevent further risk and to identify the reason for the unsteadiness. Frustratingly, the answer is usually nothing more than old age.

The nurse reappeared, equipped with her IV paraphernalia.

"Let's get labs," I said. "And the usual head CT."

As the years go by, the adult brain slowly atrophies, like a desiccated orange detaching from its rind. The shrinkage can cause problems. Cerebral veins are tethered to the superior sagittal sinus, the large blood vessel that runs front to back along the underside of the skull. As the brain contracts, these bridging veins must stretch, making them vulnerable to shearing forces caused by rapid head movements or even modest contusions. Without sufficient brain tissue to support and compress the bleeding site, small, low-pressure venous leaks may go unstanched. The blood seeps into the gap between the arachnoid membrane that encloses the brain and the lining of the skull, or dura mater. Bleeding into this space is called a subdural hematoma.

Acute subdural hematomas result from severe head trauma and expand quickly. Chronic subdural hematomas, on the other hand, often spread slowly and without visible symptoms. What really scares emergency physicians—and has me repeating to patients and their families, "Return if there's any change in behavior"—is that older people who have fallen can look fine for weeks before the bleeding causes symptoms. By then, relatives will have forgotten the long-ago head knock, attributing Granddad's confusion to the heat, the cold, or a dizzy spell. Without that critical, sometimes lifesaving clue, precious time is lost.

Forty-five minutes later, the radiologist called. "Your patient has a big subdural on the right. Evidence of old bleeding too. How is he doing?"

I was shocked. "He looked great to me. I thought the CT was a waste."

I hurried to the patient's room. The nurse was already there. "Big subdural," I said.

"Oh, gosh," she exclaimed. "Let's get him into a monitored bed."

As soon as we sat him up, the patient vomited. Nausea is a worrisome sign that increasing pressure is irritating the brain. Now I was in a hurry. If the enlarging hematoma pressed on his brain too much, the patient would suffer permanent damage.

The neurosurgeon hadn't called back. How much time had I wasted over that silly knee? I rushed upstairs and headed over to the surgery office.

"I need a neurosurgeon," I said, panting.

The secretary got on the phone. "I'll do what I can, Dr. Dajer."

No one answered her pages.

"Please keep trying," I pleaded.

Back downstairs, I found the patient tracing circles with his finger, signaling "dizzy."

"Blood pressure's going up," the nurse announced.

I started to sweat. From a hydraulics perspective, the brain is a bowl of jelly honeycombed with high-pressure pipes. Whenever blood pressure in the brain rises too much, the brain senses that it's running short on blood flow and provokes an even higher blood pressure, which in turn prompts more bleeding. "Two hours, two whole hours wasted," I kept repeating in silent self-flagellation.

Aside from surgery, there are two techniques to reduce intracranial pressure temporarily. One involves intubating the patient and giving artificial respiration. That reduces the level of carbon dioxide in the blood, which causes arteries to contract, thus shrinking overall brain volume. The second method is to give mannitol, a complex sugar, intravenously, which shrinks brain tissue by drawing water out of brain cells. Each technique buys time, and each has side effects.

"Surgery, 5025," our clerk called out.

I grabbed the handset.

"Surgery." It was the resident, not the chief surgeon.

"Listen, I've got a subdural down here," I said. "Not doing well. The on-call surgeon hasn't answered. Can you guys at least notify the OR and get things rolling?"

"Let me take a look, okay?"

Ten long minutes later, the surgeon phoned. "How are you?" he drawled, as laid-back as an airline pilot reading the altitude. "I was in the OR. Whatcha got?"

I spilled my story.

"We'll get him up," the surgeon said.

The patient stayed conscious and kept answering our questions. The old guy's brain was durable.

In the operating room, the neurosurgeon drilled four small holes in the skull, sawed between them, and lifted off a rectangle of bone the size of a credit card. The dura mater beneath was tense and black, bulging with clotted blood. The surgeon incised twice to make an X, allowed the accumulated blood to pour out, then carefully irrigated the surface of the brain while looking for signs of persistent bleeding. When everything looked good, he placed a flat rubber drain inside the incision, replaced the bone flap, stitched the scalp closed, and stapled the skin shut. Done.

Three days later, the patient was out of intensive care. Four days after that, he was in his new digs: a nursing home.

"So he did well?" the nurse asked when I gave her the follow-up.

"Amazingly," I replied. "That subdural was so big it would have killed you or me." I shook my head. "Chief complaint: two-day-old knee pain. And he looked so good. . . ."

"Don't beat yourself up." She grinned. "Around here, it's always the ones you don't worry about that you have to worry about. But that's just a nurse's opinion."

Tony Dajer is site director of the emergency division at New York Presbyterian Hospital.

CHAPTER

3

THE BOY WHO STOPPED TALKING

By Mark Cohen

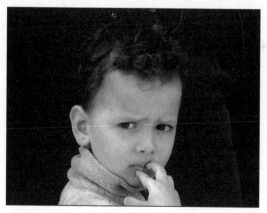

Photo 3-1

"The strangest thing about my son is that he started out talking really well, and then a couple of months ago, he just stopped."

As his mother was telling me that, the 17-month-old abandoned the toy car he had been playing with, looked at me briefly, and then toddled across my office to his mother's chair. He reached for her hand and pulled on it, insistently. She got out of her chair, and he led her over to where he had been playing. The boy took his mother's hand and placed it on top of the toy car. "Oh, the wheel fell off," she said to him, as she replaced the small plastic wheel on the axle. "Here, Mommy fixed it for you."

The boy resumed his play, rolling the car back and forth repeatedly. I watched him for a few seconds, then turned back to the mother, who now sat slumped in her chair. "He does that a lot," she said. "It's like he's just using my hand as a tool or something."

Suddenly, the boy walked back to her and climbed into her lap, putting his arms around her neck. She kissed him. "And then he's just so affectionate, like this. That's why our family doctor said that he wasn't autistic. I don't know what's wrong with him. And with my husband away, it's gotten even harder to deal with him."

The boy had been referred to me because he was not talking, and he seemed to be losing some developmental skills. That is always worrisome. As a pediatrician dealing with developmental problems, I never fail to ask if a child has lost any skills, because of the devastating possibility of a rare degenerative brain disorder like Tay-Sachs disease.

I began asking questions to review the boy's mental and motor development, keeping in mind the list of reasons for a child not to be talking by the age of 17 months. The list is long, including generalized developmental delay (the most common cause), hearing loss, and muscle coordination problems.

As I questioned her, the mother described a number of behaviors consistent with autism. Her son never turned to look at her when she called his name. He did not point at objects, either to ask for them or to call his parents' attention to them. If he saw a group of children playing, he ignored them and played on his own. He did not enjoy interactive games like peekaboo or patty-cake. He had loud tantrums for no apparent reason. He would not walk on grass or sand.

Nevertheless, if I had seen this child in the early years of my career, I would have said, as did his doctor, "He's not autistic! He's affectionate, he makes eye contact with me, he doesn't get upset if his routine is changed, and he doesn't spin around or flap his arms."

When I was in medical school and pediatric residency in the mid-1970s, I learned that autism was a brain disorder of unknown cause, that most autistic children were severely retarded, that they did not speak or interact with others, and that they were somehow locked in their own world. I was taught that if a child made eye contact with me, that meant he was not autistic.

Many of those statements, like other medical maxims I once learned, seem not to be true. We know, at least for now, that autism comprises a spectrum of brain disorders that range from mild to severe. Many children with these disorders do not show any loss of mental ability. People with autism spectrum disorders do have impaired social interaction and delayed or disordered language development and use. Some also show a pattern of atypical behaviors and activities, such as repetitive or stereotyped movements, restricted interests and preoccupations, insistence on routines, and unusual reactions to sounds, textures, or other aspects of the environment.

About 25 percent of children with autism develop language normally but then lose the ability to speak sometime between 16 and 30 months of age. The condition, called regressive autism, is not known to many physicians, so they may worry about a rare degenerative disorder instead.

We do not know exactly what causes autism spectrum disorders. Research suggests they are present from birth, although the conditions may not show up clearly until later. The cause may be a combination of a genetic predisposition—a cluster of genes that set the stage for the condition—coupled with unknown prenatal factors.

After listening to the mother's story, I tried to do a developmental assessment, a series of play-like tests and observations to see how a child is progressing in his cognitive, motor, language, and social development. But he had so little interest in the type of interactive play and socialization that is typical of children his age that I couldn't complete the assessment. This confirmed my suspicion that he was on the autism spectrum.

I looked at the mother. "What do you think about him?" I asked.

Her eyes brimmed with tears. "I think he might be autistic," she said.

"What does that mean to you?" I never assume a parent's level of understanding.

"Well, I really don't know. But I know there's something different about him." Parents of children with disabilities often have tremendous insight, a quality of knowledge we doctors ignore too often.

In the past, when I made the diagnosis of autism in a child, I was devastated. I had very little to offer the parents, who had to learn to live with a child whose mind was foreign to them. But in recent years there has been a breakthrough in the care of children with autism: the recognition that certain kinds of intervention, if initiated early—before about age 3—can produce significant improvement in the ability of many children to communicate and relate to other people.

Early intervention programs for autism focus on three areas: speech and language, behavior, and social skills. In addition, certain psychoactive medications—often in doses much smaller than those used for other patients—can help to lessen difficult behaviors. This may result from improving the child's ability to process sensory stimuli, or perhaps by reducing anxiety or other emotional reactions. In addition, groups for families and organizations like the Autism Society of America can provide information and support from experts and from parents of children with similar disabilities.

"Yes, I think you're right," I said to his mother. "There is something different about the way your son's brain works. I think that he fits into the spectrum of autism, although he doesn't fit all the characteristics of autistic children. But there are things that we can do, and that you can do, to help him grow and develop and improve."

Mark Cohen is a pediatrician in Santa Clara, California.

CHAPTER

4

WHY IS HER VISION HAZY?

By Richard Fleming

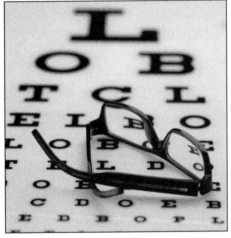

Photo 4-1

At first I thought it had to be stress. The patient was in her early forties and had been coming to my clinic for several years, complaining of weakness, stiffness when walking, numbness in her hands, occasional falls, and headaches. I ran tests the first year, including an extensive check for diabetes, anemia, and internal-organ dysfunction. All were normal. I ordered nerve conduction studies to see whether her numbness might be from carpal tunnel syndrome, which is caused by pressure on the median nerve in the wrist. They were normal. I did an echocardiogram. It was normal. I discovered that her job would be eliminated in a downsizing, and I suspected that played a major role in her complaints.

Then one Friday night, she noticed the vision in her left eye had become a bit hazy, so she came to the clinic that evening. The doctor on duty found no abnormality in either eye but thought she might have a detached retina, a true emergency and one of the few things that could get the on-call ophthalmologist to come see a patient late on a Friday night. Her retinas seemed fine, though, so he decided to see if she might have an inflamed optic nerve or a problem in her brain and ordered an MRI of her head and eye for the coming week.

The patient called me five days later to say her vision was improving and to get the results of the MRI, which had not clarified what happened. Her orbit, or eye socket, was normal. Her brain showed several small, nondescript areas that signal alterations in the white matter, the pathways along which neural impulses travel. The radiologist's report said these areas were "nonspecific and can be attributed to senescent changes." I was a little irked that the radiologist had not looked at the patient's age, which was 43. Why would a 43-year-old have "senescent changes," a throwaway term applied to the nonspecific findings that show up in our brains as we get older?

But the report did set off a question in the back of my head: Could she be in the early stages of multiple sclerosis? Optic neuritis, an inflammation of the optic nerve, could cause the visual problem. About half of all patients with optic neuritis go on to develop multiple sclerosis.

"Your MRI was pretty much normal," I hedged. "But I want you to see a neurologist for a consultation."

She pressed me to say why, so I explained that I was concerned about the possibility of MS. Like so many other illnesses, multiple sclerosis is a disease whose cause is unknown. The body's immune system attacks and destroys myelin, which is a major component of white matter. In MS, immune cells attack myelin in scattered areas, affecting the optic nerve and nerves in the brain and spinal cord. Symptoms result from delays or blockages in electrical impulses traveling down affected nerves, and problems with vision are often the first to appear. Other signs can be the loss of bladder or bowel control, difficulty walking, and heat intolerance, as well as almost any symptom of neurological dysfunction.

What leads the immune system to start attacking parts of the body itself no one knows for sure, but some evidence suggests that the response may be due to as-yet-unidentified environmental factors combined with a genetic tendency toward the disease. Multiple sclerosis occurs more frequently in the northern latitudes of Europe and the northern reaches of North America than it does closer to the equator. People born in these northern realms who move south before the age of 15 acquire the lower risk of those who were born and stayed in the south. Conversely, those born in the southern areas of Europe and North America who move to northern climes acquire the higher risk of those who were born and live in the north. Recent studies suggest that lack of sun exposure and vitamin D deficiency may play a role.

Another clue comes from genetics. It turns out that when one identical twin develops multiple sclerosis, the other has a 25 to 30 percent risk of getting it as well. For nonidentical twins and other immediate family members, the risk is 2 to 5 percent. For the population as a whole, the risk is far, far less—a tenth of a percent. Women are twice as likely as men to get it. Something genetic appears to be at work, but there must be more to the picture. One hypothesis concerns exposure to a virus or a bacterium that carries a protein similar to that in myelin. When a person with a genetic predisposition is exposed to this hypothetical virus, her immune system gets confused. It not only fights off the virus, but also begins to view the body's own myelin tissue as a foreign invader. A couple of suspect pathogens are a herpesvirus and a form of the bacterium Chlamydia.

My patient saw the neurologist several weeks later. He told her she might have multiple sclerosis, but because she had no symptoms then—her vision had cleared—there was nothing to treat. At that time, in the early 1990s, even with the possibility of illness looming in her future, there was no medication to slow the progression of the disease. The neurologist offered to do a spinal tap because an examination of the fluid surrounding the spinal cord can help make a definitive diagnosis. She declined. She accepted the fact that she might have a serious illness brewing, but watchful waiting was the only treatment option.

Seven years went by. She found a new job. Her health seemed stable, although she usually felt tired and was unable to exercise because her muscles felt weak.

Then one day she developed double vision. This can be due to the effect of multiple sclerosis on the nerve cells controlling eye movement. I sent her for another MRI, which showed much more extensive involvement of the white matter in a pattern typical of multiple sclerosis. Although the condition cannot be diagnosed based only on an MRI, a suggestive scan along with a history consistent with MS, abnormalities in the neurological exam, and the elimination of other diseases can be conclusive. There was no way to predict the course of her illness. Some patients have only occasional attacks and can go years without symptoms. Others have disabling symptoms that recur frequently.

She was started on a corticosteroid drug, which would curb the immune response in hopes of suppressing the attack on her own nerve cells. At the time this patient first started experiencing symptoms, treatment for multiple sclerosis was not very effective. The only reliable medications were steroids, which reduce inflammation during an attack. Since then, other agents have become available that can influence the course of the disease. These include interferon beta-1a, interferon beta-1b, and glatiramer acetate. By altering the body's immune response to myelin, these drugs help prevent damage to the central nervous system, thereby reducing the frequency and severity of the attacks.

Over the following year, her disease progressed rapidly, and she became confined to a wheelchair because of intractable dizziness. Her vision declined in both eyes. In an attempt to slow the progress of her illness, she was given glatiramer acetate. But the drug works best if started early in the disease, and the treatment came too late to benefit this patient. She continued her rapid decline and died of pneumonia eight years after she first developed vision problems that Friday night. Her disease had proven to be unusually severe. Most patients with multiple sclerosis have a close to normal life span.

Why did she develop multiple sclerosis? Was she a victim of having lived in northern California, and could she have avoided this illness by moving south decades earlier? There is no way she could have known sooner in life what fate had in store for her. And there is no way to know whether moving south would have made a difference.

Her daughter from out of town called me several weeks after her mother died to thank me for my care. After we talked for a few minutes, she asked if she was at increased risk for the disease. I said her risk might be slightly higher than the average, but it was still very small, and she shouldn't worry. Then I asked her where she lived.

"San Diego," she said.

"I hear it's nice down there," I responded. "You're lucky to live in such a beautiful town."

Richard Fleming is a general internist in Vallejo, California.

CHAPTER

5

INSTANT PARALYSIS WITH AN INSTANT CURE

By Frank Vertosick

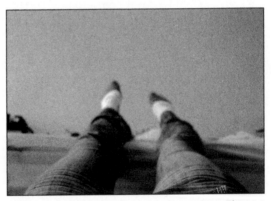

Photo 5-1

As chief of neurosurgery for a small city hospital, I've never had a phone call at 2:00 a.m. that brought me good news, and this night held true to form. The emergency room had just admitted a 22-year-old convenience store clerk, whom I will call Rachel. She had awakened several hours earlier with a rather annoying problem: she could not move her legs. According to the ER physician, Rachel noticed that she could not roll over in bed and, when the fog of sleep finally cleared, discovered that she had two lifeless logs where her lower extremities used to be.

She lived alone and, not wishing to disturb her parents living miles away, managed to crawl to her nightstand and phone directly for an ambulance. When I arrived, Rachel was still strapped to a spinal board, the right sleeve of her nightgown rolled up to allow for the intravenous line.

"Does anything hurt?" I asked.

"No," she said, shrugging. "I really feel fine . . . except for this leg thing."

"Are they numb?" I continued, stroking her bare shins with my index finger.

"Nah, I feel that. They just feel funny, you know, heavy. Do you think this is serious? When can I go home? I have to open the store at six." She smiled. "Gotta make the coffee!"

Further interrogation revealed little. Rachel was healthy, no illnesses, no medications, no surgeries. A smoker since age 14, she used marijuana sporadically, but there was no other history of drug use. No traumas, no chance of pregnancy (her boyfriend had abruptly dumped her six months earlier, and she still seethed when discussing him), no history of depression or other mental illness, no significant family history. She was in good health. Except for the "leg thing."

In addition to lacking any obvious pathology, she also lacked health insurance. The ER had already set up an MRI of her entire spine and summoned the technician from home to do it. This might yield an answer—but I suspected the truth about her condition already, and I was reluctant to saddle this poor woman with thousands of dollars of expensive pictures. The tests would all be negative anyway.

A quick examination confirmed my suspicions. When I poked her foot with a pin, she yelped but didn't move her legs. Yet her reflexes were normal, and the tone of her leg muscles was good. Finally, her Babinski sign—a neural reflex that causes the big toe to go down when the sole of the foot is stroked—was normal. These findings, coupled with a blasé attitude toward her paralysis (a mental state known in neurology as "la belle indifférence"), made me suspect a rather distasteful diagnosis: hysteria.

The word "hysteria" derives from the Greek word for womb, and for centuries the condition was thought to be a feminine affliction arising from bad uterine humors. Women hysterics outnumber men six to one for reasons yet unknown. What is known is that the womb plays no role. Many neurological conditions, including migraines and multiple sclerosis, afflict women disproportionately. The ovaries and the hormones they produce or the double X chromosomes are more likely culprits.

Today, hysteria is known by the more palatable but still inaccurate moniker "conversion disorder." It manifests acutely in the form of blindness, paralysis, or even coma, with no apparent organic disease. Sigmund Freud believed that the hysterical mind converts some psychic trauma into a physical malady that will both garner sympathy and allow the sufferer to hide from her problems behind a shield of illness. Decades before Freud, the great French neurologist Jean-Martin Charcot suggested that hysteria was indeed an organic brain illness, not the product of a disturbed or demon-possessed mind, but Freud's explanation gained wider acceptance.

Although many hysterics complain of mental distress (like Rachel's boyfriend woes), recent neurophysiological evidence from PET scans and functional MRIs suggests that the malady may be akin to a seizure initiated by the frontal lobes, and so is a condition of the brain as well as the mind. Some people may have a vulnerability to this kind of response to stress. Thus Charcot was probably right (he usually was), and Freud was probably wrong (no surprise there either).

The cardinal sign of hysteria—indifference to an obviously crippling neurological predicament—is not entirely reliable. I once cared for a teenager who was suddenly struck blind. Because she seemed apathetic about her condition, she was mistakenly given a diagnosis of hysteria. In fact, she was both blind and apathetic because of a brain tumor. Nevertheless, indifference is still a useful clue, particularly when the physical examination is normal. Rachel's preserved reflexes, good leg tone, downward Babinski sign, and preserved sensation were all inconsistent with known organic causes of sudden paraplegia (paralysis in both legs). Her lack of pain also made other causes like a ruptured disk, brain hemorrhage, or spinal abscess highly unlikely. Her nonchalance was simply icing on the diagnostic cake.

Conversion paralysis is very different from willful malingering because the hysterical patients really believe they cannot move. I have seen inexperienced physicians, anxious to expose a faker, injure people by placing clamps on their fingers or plunging needles deep into thigh muscles, only to be astounded and mortified when patients make no attempt to pull away. So I was gentle with Rachel, both physically and verbally.

I told her that most likely nothing serious was going on and that she probably had a "vitamin deficiency." I instructed the nurses to infuse a liter of intravenous nutrients. The solution's impressive amber hue suggests to the patient that some "real medicine" is being administered. This is one aspect of hysterical paralysis that still smacks of a psychiatric origin: patients must be convinced that they are being treated as if they have an organic disease. Simply telling them they are imagining things doesn't work very well.

There is an old adage: Neurology is what you do while you are waiting for the film to be developed. Physicians rely too heavily on imaging machines, and I saw no urgent need for scanning this patient. Her examination and history told her story well enough. True, the doctor must always rule out physical illness before diagnosing conversion syndrome, but in Rachel's case, infusing some vitamins could be done in the time it took to fire up a cold MRI machine. By then I would know.

Twenty minutes after the infusion ended, Rachel's legs roared to life, and she walked out the door. I went home, tired but happy in the knowledge that I hadn't allowed a single freakish spasm of a young woman's brain to land her in the poorhouse or in the psychiatric ward.

Frank Vertosick Jr., MD, is the author of Why We Hurt *and* The Genius Within.

CHAPTER

6

WHY DOES HER BELLY HURT?

By Tony Dajer

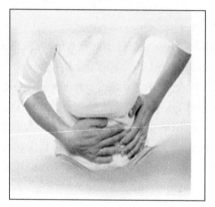

Photo 6-1

Everyone in the emergency room froze. Following the screams, I hurried to a far cubicle.

"Oh my God," a woman shrieked, clutching her belly. She looked to be about 40, was noticeably overweight, and was wearing a business suit.

"You okay?" I whispered to the attending physician.

She nodded and said: "She had a gastric bypass two years ago. Sudden onset of severe epigastric pain. Her chest X-ray shows no free air. We're on our way to a CT scan."

Air in the abdomen equals stomach or intestinal perforation, but it doesn't always show up on an X-ray. Although perforation is rare in healthy young women, her bypass for weight loss put her in another category. I tried to think up a list of likely complications, but I couldn't come up with more than a few.

"You'll be okay," I said and grabbed the stretcher railing.

"Ow. Oh, Jesus," she said, gasping as we headed down the hall. "I can't believe this."

The attending physician turned to a nurse: "Six of morphine IV, please."

A half hour later we had a diagnosis.

"The scan shows free air. Her surgeon wants her uptown," the attending physician said. "He did the bypass."

One out of 20 American adults is severely obese, 5 of those 20 are obese, and another 7 are overweight. The categories are not arbitrary. A mathematical computation called the body mass index uses weight and height to calculate risk (see www.cdc.gov/nccdphp/dnpa/bmi/calc-bmi.htm). If your body mass index hits 40, you are severely obese—something like a 5-foot-4-inch woman weighing 230 pounds. Between 1986 and 2000, the percentage of Americans who qualify as severely obese quadrupled. The statistics go on and on: a severely obese 25-year-old will die 12 years earlier than normal; obesity illnesses devour more than 50 billion dollars a year in medical costs in the United States.

Although exercise and diet can clearly control obesity in the vast majority of cases, an increasing number of people are turning to bariatric surgery. In 1998 American doctors performed 13,365 such surgeries. In 2004 the estimate went up to 140,000. For emergency room doctors, the numbers are even scarier, because we will see about 40 percent of those patients within three years.

To understand what I was facing, I turned to Howard Beaton, an old friend and chief of surgery at a nearby hospital. Before 9/11, both of us carried some extra pounds. On that terrible day, in our emergency room four blocks from the World Trade Center, he directed surgeons on dozens of trauma cases while I coordinated the rest of the emergency department. The shock of it all set us both on the road to fitness. I started jogging; he ran on a treadmill during nights on call. Four and a half years later he remains slim, almost gaunt.

"I started doing bariatric surgery in 2003," he said as we walked into his operating room. "It is extraordinary. I've had patients who married, who started working again. One became a policeman. When they go for months between visits, you often don't recognize them. A completely unimagined person emerges."

Lying on the table in front of us is a 5-foot-2-inch 220-pound woman. Beaton draws his scalpel from the lower edge of her sternum to a point two inches above her belly button. "I used to make an incision down to here," he says, indicating a spot six inches lower. "Now, this much is plenty. Bariatric surgery has a steep learning curve."

Beaton slices through a hefty layer of globular, canary yellow fat and enters the peritoneum, the membrane that lines the abdominal cavity. Coils of pink, wormy intestine appear. Beaton uses a modified version of an operation devised by surgeon Cesar Roux a century ago for other conditions. He will divide the stomach, leaving a very small pouch attached to the esophagus and the rest connected to the small intestine.

He severs the intestine below the stomach, then burns a hole in the intestine three feet down. Out come a menacing pair of stapler guns to connect the stomach portion to that opening. The next step is to drastically limit food access to the stomach. He applies his two staple rows across the stomach and cuts between them, dividing the stomach. He has now created a small pouch connected to the esophagus. The bulk of the stomach and duodenum never see food again.

"I tell patients their stomach is now about the size of an egg," he explains.

Finally, to link the newly shrunken stomach to working intestine, he brings up the still-severed section of intestine, makes a hole in the stomach pouch, and zips the two together.

"Amazing," I mutter.

Beaton turns to me and asks, "Aren't those staplers something?"

The first weight-loss operation took place in 1954. Designed to prevent food absorption by connecting the near end of the small intestine to the far, it ultimately caused too much malnutrition and, for reasons unknown, liver cirrhosis. In the 1960s surgeons developed the gastric bypass, which remains the mainstay in the United States. In the 1980s the practice of limiting food capacity by stapling the stomach nearly all the way across became available. Although it seemed like a simple solution, the staple lines tended to come apart.

More recently, in Europe and Australia, stomach banding has gained favor. In that procedure, a saline-filled collar is fastened around the upper stomach and then filled or emptied through tubing connected to a port under the skin. Approved by the FDA in 2001, its attraction is its simplicity, especially if done laparoscopically. Its principal drawback is that patients might lose less weight than with the current standard procedure, known as the Roux-en-Y bypass. That is why American surgeons still perform bypasses in four out of five cases. The largest study to date shows that bariatric surgery reduces excess weight by 61 percent and cures sleep apnea, hypertension, and diabetes in more than two-thirds of patients.

"For diabetics," Beaton says, "the effect is so fast we stop their pills on discharge, or their sugars will bottom out."

A Canadian study of morbidly obese patients found that there were proportionally fewer deaths among patients who had gastric bypass surgery than there were among those who did not: 0.7 percent of the bypass group died within five years, as opposed to 6.2 percent of the control group. Impressive, but there are problems too. Huge battles loom over insurance coverage. Depending on the procedure, it may run up to $30,000 and require a three-day hospital stay.

"Some plans require six months of documented attempts at medically supervised weight loss before approving surgery," says Beaton, shaking his head. "Which means you're taking people who already consider themselves failures and setting them up to fail again."

And experience counts for the surgeon. One study of the banding technique showed that a surgeon's first 30 patients had a 37 percent complication rate, the next 30, only 7 percent.

Constant practice is even more important: Surgeons doing less than one case a month lost one in 20 patients. Their more prolific colleagues lost one in 300.

The overall death rate from the different procedures is 0.1 percent for banding and 0.5 percent for bypass. Darkening that picture is a new study of 16,155 Medicare patients, in which 4.6 percent of patients died within a year of the operation. Medicare patients tend to be older and more disabled, but the results give pause.

"These patients are inherently high risk," Beaton says. "As an ER doctor, you need to know that with post-op complications, your clinical exam is almost worthless. I've seen huge abscesses in patients with no abdominal tenderness or fever. When they present with abdominal pain, they almost always need a CT scan. One pitfall of the Roux-en-Y is that it creates the potential for internal hernias [ruptures] that can trap loops of intestine and cut off blood flow. Then, as opposed to the bowel obstructions that we're used to where it is reasonable to suction the stomach and wait, you'd better operate immediately."

The list of possible complications is daunting: bleeding, blood clots in the lungs, gastric-pouch rupture, post-op vomiting, infection, scarring that narrows the intestine, ulcers, gallstones, abdominal-wall hernias, and iron and vitamin deficiencies.

Beaton says, "The best rule is, when these patients get sick, diagnose them fast and go right in when necessary."

As for our patient, her surgeon explained that she had developed an opening, or ulcer, where the intestine was stapled to the stomach pouch. "Unusual two years out," he said. "We went in and patched it up. She did fine."

I can't help wondering how many cases like hers are yet to come.

Tony Dajer is site director of the emergency division at New York Presbyterian Hospital.

CHAPTER

7

A SLEEPY SECRET

By Tony Dajer

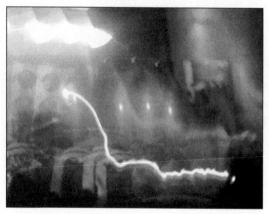

Photo 7-1

The woman burst through the emergency room doors, shouting: "Where's my son?"

"Over here," I blurted, startled by her entrance. Short and wiry, she flew past the paramedics to her motionless, well-built 25-year-old. Then, turning to me, she rose on the balls of her feet and hissed, "I told those doctors he needed an MRI!"

"Does he have epilepsy, ma'am?" I asked carefully. "Any type of seizure disorder?"

"He did this once before," she continued, as if not listening. "Those idiots upstate couldn't tell me what was wrong. Three months ago he had this . . . event. Same as today. They told us to see a neurologist. But the damn insurance company wouldn't approve the MRI."

Trying to take control of the situation, I pulled aside the lead paramedic. "Tell me again—why did you intubate him?"

"He was comatose," the burly man in the blue uniform said. "Didn't respond to Narcan" —an antidote to overdoses of opiates, like heroin—"then he started seizing."

"Full-blown seizures?" I asked.

"Hard to tell," the paramedic replied, wiping his forehead. "Jerking his arms back and forth, not breathing well. We decided not to wait, so we sedated him—that stopped the seizures—and then we put the tube in."

Comatose patients have a tendency to vomit stomach contents into their lungs. A cuffed breathing tube prevents that. "Sounds reasonable," I said. "And when the family called 911, what exactly did they say?"

"Mom found him in bed, couldn't wake him up."

The young man on the gurney looked utterly peaceful—except for the plastic breathing tube arcing out of his mouth. I turned back to the mother and asked, "Did he have a CAT scan that first time?"

She smirked. "It came out normal."

A young woman came over to where we were standing. "I'm his sister," she said.

Seeing a new opportunity for information, I asked, "Any drugs that you know of? Medications?"

Mother and daughter's heads both shook an emphatic no. "He's a good boy. No drinking, no craziness," Mom cut in.

"He had some friends over last night. They hung out upstairs," the sister added. "Maybe a few beers. Nothing more."

The young man's physical exam offered no clues. His vital signs were perfect; his pupils were small but reacted well to light; his arms and legs barely moved when pinched, but they had good tone, not the flaccid splay of paralysis. I went down the differential diagnosis. Drug overdose? That would have been detected three months earlier, the first time this happened. Brain bleed or meningitis? Obviously these were the nastiest contenders, but my alarm bells weren't going off; coma aside, Doug looked too good. Persistent seizures? He lay inert as a statue (although it is possible for a brain to have epileptic electrical activity yet cause no visible muscle contractions).

The best clue I had was that this event was a repeat. But a repeat of what? Relapsing encephalitis? Narcolepsy? A degenerative neuronal disorder? A new form of mad cow disease? I envisioned the answer buried in some thick tome titled *Neurological Disorders You Can't Even Imagine*.

Doug's mother grabbed my arm. "What is wrong with him?" she pleaded, tears now welling up.

"Don't worry. We'll do the tests he needs."

A CAT scan showed nothing (again). Minutes later, Doug started thrashing and breathing quickly, as if the breathing tube were gagging him. Good sign. Was he waking up? I deflated the cuff and pulled the tube. Coughing until he turned red, he tried to sit up, popped his eyes open, then fell back. Abruptly he resumed breathing very quickly, stopped for a full minute, then revved up again.

"Is that Cheyne-Stokes breathing?" the nurse asked me. This ragged, stop-and-start breathing pattern—so distinctive it has its own eponym—indicates a malfunction in the brain stem's breathing center. I had seen it most recently in a patient with lupus-induced brain inflammation. He had died.

The toxicology screen came back clean: no alcohol, no Valium, no cocaine. And the rest of Doug's blood work was stone-cold normal. Stumped, I phoned a member of the intensive care team. "Twenty-five-year-old man," I began. "Unexplained coma, maybe seizures. Might need a spinal tap. On the positive side, neck's supple, no fever, no white count. Either way, he needs to be in the ICU."

"Okay," the junior resident said. "But please call our attending. She has to approve."

Two minutes later I had the attending on the phone. "Sara here."

"Sorry to sound so vague," I said, then recapped the story.

Silence on the other end. Finally she asked, "Is this kid on GHB?"

"Family denies drugs," I said, instantly hearing how weak that sounded. "Idiot!" I thought. "I'll call you back," I answered aloud. I wanted to slam down the receiver.

I cornered Mom and sister. "Sorry, but we have to know this: Did Doug do GHB last night?"

Mom did a double take: "What?" But a look flitted across the sister's face.

"Please ask his friends specifically. Tell them it's life-or-death."

Gamma hydroxybutyrate (commonly called G, liquid ecstasy, Georgia home boy, or cherry meth) is to rave parties of the new millennium what cocaine was to Wall Street of the 1980s. A natural brain neurotransmitter, GHB is a stimulant in small doses. Take an extra hit and it is said to bring on a warm, dreamy feeling, with some sexual arousal thrown in for good measure. As a recreational drug, it enhances the hypnotic, techno-music-driven, quivering state that defines rave parties.

The catch? At higher concentrations GHB binds to the GABA brain receptors, just as Valium does. This interaction produces GHB's signature effect: lights out, like walking into a Mike Tyson uppercut. Worse, GHB's dose effect is wildly unpredictable. A tad too much and you can go from life of the party to 911 emergency. (GHB was used as an anesthetic in the 1960s, but was discontinued precisely because dosing was so touchy.) Little wonder that it has become a leading cause of drug-induced coma and ranks second among all illegal drugs in requiring emergency consultations. Throw in alcohol—which competes for the same liver enzymes that metabolize GHB—and the duration and severity of the drug's effects zoom off the charts.

Side effects of GHB overdose run the gamut from vomiting, muscle spasms, and seizures to slow heart rate and cardiac arrest. Since its rise in popularity in the 1990s, GHB has killed hundreds. And it is highly addictive: Some abusers need a hit every two hours. Withdrawal after chronic use is particularly nasty. Delirium and life-threatening agitation can flare for weeks after GHB is stopped.

GHB has also gained notoriety as the "date-rape drug." An odorless, colorless liquid easily masked by a cocktail, it is quickly metabolized and not detectable in routine blood and urine tests. A specialized lab might pick it up, but only by analyzing an immediately obtained urine sample. GHB doesn't even have to knock a victim out. At a sub-KO dose it can induce amnesia, arousal, and a passive, compliant state of mind.

The sister returned. "The friends 'fessed up," she said with a brisk, grim nod. "They did some GHB last night."

Mom just stared. Then her shoulders sagged.

I called Sara back. "Bingo. And thanks for turning my brain back on. That 'second episode' malarkey had me going."

"You're welcome," she replied graciously. "My husband's a cop. He's seen a lot of it lately."

I turned back to the family. The fight with the insurance company over getting an MRI? The kid watching his mom go to the mat for him—for a lie? Then doing it all over again?

I raised my eyebrows at the sister. Her gaze went opaque. Who knew what went on here? I wondered.

The good news was that Doug didn't display any signs of chronic GHB use, and once this dose of the drug was out of his system, he would be none the worse for wear.

"He should wake up in a few hours," I reassured his mother. "He'll be okay."

"No, he won't," she muttered, her voice fierce again.

Tony Dajer is site director of the emergency division at New York Presbyterian Hospital.

CHAPTER

8

WHAT IS FANNING HIS TEMPER?

By Ronald Schouten

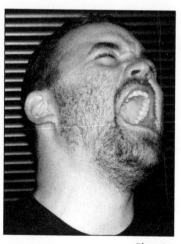

Photo 8-1

Bill, a managing partner of a prominent local law firm, frequently used me as a psychiatric consultant for the firm's personnel issues. So I wasn't surprised to get a call from him about his partner, Steve. We had spoken about Steve several times in just the past year. This time, Bill sounded desperate.

"He's finally done it," Bill said. "I just have two questions for you. First, what the hell is wrong with him? And second, can it be fixed? If not, he'll have to leave the firm. We've had enough."

Brilliant, demanding, and aggressive, Steve had been terrifying associates and support staff for as long as anyone could remember. He was kept on because he brought in lots of work and because he was a valuable mentor.

This time, the problem was something Steve had done outside the office. Running late for court, he had run a red light. When he saw flashing blue lights in his rearview mirror, he just drove faster, stopping only when another police car pulled in front of him. Officers approached his car, one with his weapon drawn. Steve, who handled a good deal of litigation for the city, immediately began yelling at them.

"Don't you know who I am?" he demanded to know. "I'm the guy the mayor turns to for legal advice when you clowns get yourselves into trouble. What the f--- are you stopping me for? I'm due in court." One of the officers tersely explained the illegality of running the red light, reckless driving, speeding, and failing to stop. Steve took the ticket and drove off, cursing and vowing to get the officer fired.

Word of the encounter quickly spread. Confronted by Bill, Steve admitted that he had mouthed off to the police officers, but claimed that he had every right to do so. Bill told Steve he needed to take two weeks off and get a psychiatric evaluation, or lose his job. That's when Bill called me.

In my role as a psychiatric consultant on workplace behavioral health matters, I'm often asked to evaluate people whose behavior is about to cost them their jobs. The person being evaluated is always a key source of information, but evaluations of fitness for duty and disability also require more objective reports.

So I asked Steve's law partners what they thought was going on. They reported that Steve had always been tough on people, but there had been a turn for the worse in the past few years. He was more irritable, more abrupt, and no longer seemed to enjoy his work. Clients had asked if Steve was having health problems, saying he just wasn't himself and seemed forgetful. With that information in hand, as well as complete physical and laboratory work from Steve's primary care physician, I was ready to see him.

Entering my office, Steve was an imposing guy. He stood six feet tall, with a thick neck and a bit of a paunch—the build of the aging college football lineman that he was. He was defiant and disdainful of the process. His description of events was peppered with words like "nonsense," "bullsh--," and "stupid," and he expressed dismay that he was now being forced to see a "shrink." He insisted nothing was wrong. "I've always been a hard-ass," he said. "That's just my style. And no one ever complained before."

"So, what's changed?" I asked.

Steve grudgingly acknowledged that things had gotten worse over the past three years. Assertive and demanding by nature, in the past he had felt in control of his world. Now he was always on edge and prone to emotional outbursts. He was exhausted and had lost his motivation. He no longer enjoyed doing things he used to enjoy, a symptom known as anhedonia—Greek for "lack of pleasure." He was more forgetful and not as accurate or productive as he had been, but he wondered if this was just a result of turning 55.

WHAT FLIPPED THE SWITCH?

It seemed clear that Steve's surly and aggressive behavior reflected more than just an unpleasant disposition. A number of physical illnesses can cause such deteriorations in behavior. Leading contenders, alone and in combination, include endocrine disorders like thyroid disease and diabetes, cardiac disease, infectious diseases, neurological conditions, and cancer. But Steve's primary care physician had given him a clean bill of health, other than moderate hypertension and a 20-pound weight gain over the past several years.

Next on my list was substance abuse, which is notorious for contributing to problematic behaviors. But Steve denied using illegal drugs, misusing prescription medications, or drinking excessively. His physical exam and lab work were consistent with this, as were his partners' reports.

With the obvious physical illnesses and substance abuse ruled out, it was time to consider psychiatric disorders. It was possible that Steve had a personality disorder—a long-standing, maladaptive pattern of experiencing and interacting with the rest of the world. Steve's interactions with me, the reports from his partners, and his history were all consistent with a personality disorder, or at least a worrisome exacerbation of some very negative personality traits.

But Steve's personality had been the same since he was in college. While his aggressiveness didn't necessarily make him a pleasant guy, it had served him well professionally. He also had friends and a wife of many years. So the evidence for a full-blown personality disorder was not strong. I needed to focus on what could have caused an exacerbation of his pre-existing traits.

While several psychiatric problems, including depression, might explain Steve's worsening behavior, his irritability, sad mood, decreased energy, and difficulty sleeping weren't severe enough to make a conclusive diagnosis.

TOO LITTLE AIR

It was with the exploration of Steve's sleep problem that things got interesting. Sleep deprivation can have many physical and mental effects, including impaired cognitive and physical performance, increased errors, decreased immune response, and changes in mood.

Disturbed sleep can be both a symptom and a cause of conditions such as depression, bipolar disorder, and changes in personality similar to Steve's. In some studies, brain scans of severely sleep-deprived individuals are similar to those of psychopaths, people with an extreme form of antisocial personality disorder.

So I asked Steve about his sleeping. He fell asleep just fine, he said, but was restless during the night and woke up feeling unrested, usually with a headache.

"Do you snore?" I asked.

"Let's put it this way," Steve said. "I've had people pound on the walls of hotel rooms at night complaining that I was keeping them awake."

"Does your wife ever notice that you stop breathing while you are sleeping?"

"She flips out when that happens and pokes me to make sure I'm still alive."

Steve was describing classic symptoms of sleep apnea, a condition in which a person either stops breathing entirely or has impaired airflow while sleeping, depriving the brain, and the rest of the body, of oxygen. Sleep apnea can cause hypertension, vascular problems, and cognitive and behavioral changes.

In the most common form of sleep apnea, obstructive sleep apnea, the upper airway becomes blocked as muscles relax during sleep; air being forced over the obstruction causes snoring. A variety of factors can cause the condition, including having a short, thick neck, gaining weight, and using substances that cause excessive sleepiness, like medications or alcohol.

Not everyone with obstructive sleep apnea looks like Steve, but his physique fit the classic profile. Sleep apnea moved up on my list of possible diagnoses.

Steve's primary care physician agreed to send Steve for a polysomnogram, an overnight study in a sleep laboratory in which the patient's airflow, oxygen levels, muscle movements, heart rhythm, and brain waves are monitored. Steve expressed skepticism that he would be able to sleep in a strange place connected to all those machines. But he fell asleep easily and woke up only when the technician entered the room when his oxygen saturation level had repeatedly dropped to 85 percent.

The technician had Steve put on a breathing mask connected to a machine that generates air pressure, helping to keep the airway open. This therapy, called continuous positive airway pressure, or CPAP, ensures that the brain gets enough oxygen. With CPAP in place, Steve's oxygen saturation was fine. The sleep specialist recommended that Steve continue the treatment at home, and also that he lose some weight and avoid alcohol at bedtime.

Two weeks later, Steve told me he had started feeling better almost immediately. He awoke feeling rested, his headaches were gone, and he felt more on top of things. His wife had even commented that he was calmer and less irritable.

I recommended that Steve return to work. I warned Bill that treatment for sleep apnea would not necessarily reverse Steve's habit of treating others poorly, but it would give him more control over his behavior. I was hopeful that with clear expectations set on his behavior, the firm would see a new and improved Steve.

My hopes proved to be justified. Six months later, Steve's mind was clearer, his work had improved, and he was back to mentoring the younger attorneys and serving his clients.

Ronald Schouten is director of the Law & Psychiatry Service of the Massachusetts General Hospital and associate professor of psychiatry at Harvard Medical School, as well as co-author of Almost a Psychopath *(2012).*

CHAPTER

9

WHY IS SHE GETTING THINNER?

By Douglas G. Adler

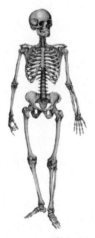

Photo 9-1

Our first patient in the gastroenterology clinic one morning was a 68-year-old retired cafeteria worker with vague abdominal pains. Basic blood tests and an endoscopic examination of her digestive tract turned up nothing, so she was referred to me for further evaluation. The pains in her mid-abdomen came and went, sometimes radiated to other areas, and were often triggered by meals. Some days she had no pain. She often felt better when fasting or after a bowel movement.

My first thought was that the patient might have irritable bowel syndrome, a condition that is associated with intermittent abdominal pain in the absence of any visible abnormality. But it would be unusual for it to turn up for the first time in a woman this age.

I noticed that the patient was quite thin, 5 feet 4 inches tall, and only 100 pounds. When I asked her if she had lost any weight, she simply shrugged and told me she didn't even own a scale. I asked to look at the photo on her driver's license for comparison, and she did appear to have shed some pounds. Still, when I performed a physical examination, she seemed healthy.

Her chart showed that she was taking an oral medication to lower the level of glucose in the blood. I asked her if she was diabetic.

"Yes, I am," she replied. "It was just diagnosed a few months ago, much to my surprise."

"Why were you surprised by the diagnosis?" I asked.

"I never had problems with my blood sugar until now," she said. "Plus, nobody in my family has diabetes, so I guess I was just the lucky one. Now they tell me I have to take these medicines forever, and I hate checking my blood sugar all day long!"

The fact that she had new-onset diabetes raised a red flag for me, especially because she was so thin. Diabetes that develops after childhood is often a disease of overweight individuals who have become resistant to insulin, the hormone the pancreas secretes to lower the level of glucose in the bloodstream. This type of diabetes is uncommon in thin people.

"Does the pain in your stomach ever radiate through to your back?" I asked.

"Yes, yes, it does," she said after thinking for a moment. "Sometimes when I lie down at night."

"We need to take a look in your belly and make sure your pancreas is okay," I told her. "I'll order a CT scan of your abdomen right away."

The pancreas, which sits behind the stomach and in front of the spine, is a woefully misunderstood organ. Most of us think that the stomach is the main digestive organ, but in fact it does only a small part of the job. The pancreas secretes enzymes that break down foods into their basic building blocks. These simple sugars, fats, and peptides are then absorbed by the small intestine, whereas the colon primarily absorbs water. Most people are blissfully unaware of the pancreas until it gets them into trouble, usually by becoming inflamed, a condition known as pancreatitis, or by turning cancerous.

Vague abdominal pains are a dime a dozen, but vague abdominal pains in the presence of new-onset diabetes raise the possibility of pancreatic cancer. In addition, abdominal pain that radiates to the back often suggests a problem in the pancreas itself.

Despite intense investigation over the past decade, the relationship between diabetes and pancreatic cancer remains poorly understood. Many patients with pancreatic cancer develop high blood sugar, or hyperglycemia, which can progress to full-fledged diabetes. The reasons for this remain unknown. One hypothesis is that tumors of the pancreas destroy enough of the insulin-producing islet cells in the pancreas to cause diabetes. Another possibility is that pancreatic tumors somehow make patients become insensitive to insulin. The basis for this hypothesis is that patients often regain sensitivity to insulin following the removal of the tumor.

Some physicians have advocated studying patients with new-onset diabetes as a population at high risk for pancreatic cancer. They have proposed screening these patients with special blood tests, ultrasound exams, and CT scans. However, there are reasons to be cautious. More than one million new cases of diabetes are diagnosed in the United States each year, but pancreatic cancer is comparatively rare, with only about 30,000 new cases in the United States during the same period of time. Testing everyone who developed diabetes in hopes of finding a small number of patients with pancreatic cancer would be prohibitively costly.

Still, if the diabetes leads to the discovery of the cancer (and not the other way around), the cancer is more likely to be at a stage at which it can be successfully removed. Understanding this possibility is especially important because the overwhelming majority of patients have their pancreatic cancer diagnosed when the cancer has become incurable. Most patients die within six months of diagnosis. Usually the tumor has already spread to another organ, or the primary tumor has wrapped itself around one of the nearby major abdominal arteries, making surgical removal of the tumor too risky.

Later that day I got the results of the patient's CT scan. It showed fullness in her pancreas that could be a tumor. She was hospitalized for further testing.

The next morning, I performed an endoscopic ultrasound. After the patient was sedated, I inserted an endoscope with a tiny built-in ultrasound instrument through her mouth and into her stomach and intestines. The ultrasound let me look through the wall of her stomach and small intestine and see her pancreas in exquisite detail. What had appeared as fullness on the CT scan looked like a classic pancreatic cancer. To confirm the diagnosis, I inserted a needle through the endoscope to take a biopsy from the core of the mass. A pathologist standing by examined the tissue and verified that the cells from the mass were cancerous. The tumor was surgically removed the following week.

My patient was lucky. If she had waited a few more months to get medical attention, she might have died from inoperable pancreatic cancer.

The relationship between diabetes and pancreatic cancer is still being explored, and doctors must rely on their clinical judgment and experience when deciding which patients with new-onset diabetes should be screened for pancreatic cancer. Yet, given how few tools exist for discovering patients with pancreatic cancer early in the course of the illness, any new way to identify potentially curable patients is a source of hope.

Douglas G. Adler is assistant professor of medicine at the University of Texas Medical School at Houston.

CHAPTER

10

A STRESS CASE OR
A SERIOUS DISEASE?

By Robert A. Norman

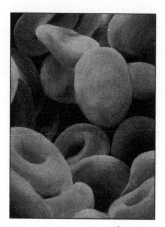

Photo 10-1

Mary was waiting for me in the examination room. A mildly plump 55-year-old, she looked at me nervously as I came in, waiting for her chance to spill out all her aches and pains and concerns. "Hello, Mary," I said. "How have you been?"

"Not so good," she replied, handing me a sheet of paper with a long list of medications written on it.

I had seen Mary many times over the last five years in my dermatology office, so I was no stranger to her lists or her wide variety of ailments, real and imagined. During the last visit, her chief complaint had been irritated sores on the scalp. At the time, she told me she was compulsive and kept scratching the sores until they bled—a classic sign of neurodermatitis, a condition in which a person scratches the skin repeatedly, usually to relieve stress or tension. We see it quite often in our practice, and from talking to Mary I knew she had enough stress in her life to sink a ship.

I prescribed a cortisone solution for two weeks and an over-the-counter product containing castor oil and menthol that cooled the sores on her scalp. I also recommended relaxation techniques and counseling, which often help with neurodermatitis, but our subsequent conversations left me with the impression that Mary hadn't taken my advice.

I looked at the list of medications that she had written down—Prozac, clonazepam, and others, mostly treatments for depression and stress-induced disorders. Included on the paper were small written comments and questions: "Calcium citrate caps—should I take these or not?" and "Need to take this in the morning" next to her Prozac. Over the years she had suffered from a number of other problems as well: tonsillitis, mono, urinary tract infections, blisters, mouth sores and chapped lips, acne, and high cholesterol. The constellation of symptoms and conditions painted a picture of a stressed person who was chronically taxing her immune system. She seemed to be fighting hard to stay above water.

Now Mary had a new skin-related complaint. "Over the last year I get these bruises all over me," she told me. "They just appear out of nowhere and itch badly." Knowing her previous history, I had to consider the strong possibility that stress was influencing her symptoms. When I asked her if she was experiencing increased anxiety, she was very candid, mentioning that she was having marital problems. She also said that the sores on her scalp had returned and that she was suffering from depression. When I asked if she had any trouble breathing—something that often accompanied her severe bouts of anxiety—she said yes.

With that information in mind, I proceeded to the physical examination. When I looked at her legs, I noticed she had petechiae, red and purple pinpoint-size dots caused by a minor hemorrhage from broken capillary blood vessels. Petechiae can be a side effect of aspirin use. Infections can lead to petechiae, which are also associated with alcoholism, AIDS, vasculitis (an inflammation of the blood vessels), and certain cancers such as leukemia or lymphoma. Another reason for petechiae is thrombocytopenia, a shortage of blood platelets. Also called thrombocytes, platelets are cells about 10 percent the diameter of red blood cells and are responsible for forming the clots that stop bleeding.

Mary also had small purple bruises on her arms and legs, called purpura, brought on by bleeding under the skin. Together the purpura and petechiae signaled to me that Mary could be suffering from something far more serious than her previous bouts with neurodermatitis and other ailments.

I ordered some tests, including a complete blood count, platelets, urinalysis, and thyroid and chemistry profiles and prescribed the medicines that helped relieve her scalp itch after her last visit.

When Mary's lab tests came back, some of the results were abnormal, including a small amount of blood in her urine, but what really jumped out was her platelet count. A normal count is 150,000 to 450,000 per microliter of blood. Mary's was less than 20,000.

For two weeks my team and I worked to exclude a long list of conditions that can result in blood abnormalities. We had to test Mary for leukemia, HIV, hepatitis C, lupus, cirrhosis, and medication problems, among others. After gathering all the data, we came to a diagnosis of idiopathic (meaning "cause unknown") thrombocytopenic purpura, or ITP. Although it is poorly understood, the main culprit in ITP is believed to be an autoimmune response. While your immune system normally protects your body from disease and infection, in ITP, for unknown reasons, it attacks and destroys its own platelets. The adult population with ITP, a chronic and noninfectious disease, numbers approximately 100,000 in the United States, with women outnumbering men three to two.

Not only can ITP result in petechiae and bruising, but if the platelet count falls below 30,000, patients might experience bleeding from the nostrils and gums and into the urine and stool. If a person has a very low count, less than 10,000, she runs a high risk of hematomas (pools of blood outside the vessels) in the mouth or on other moist tissues and extensive bleeding from small cuts or abrasions. Below 10,000, fatal complications can also result from brain hemorrhages, spontaneous gastrointestinal bleeding, or other internal bleeding if any trauma occurs.

During the time I worked with Mary, her blood platelet count dropped to 1,000, a medical emergency. She was hospitalized several times, given transfusions of platelets twice, and treated with high doses of the steroid prednisone, which can raise the blood platelet count.

A hematologist colleague and I discussed Mary's case several times, and the drama of her ever-lowering platelet count pushed us in the direction of recommending more aggressive intervention—removal of the spleen. That fist-size organ helps fight infection and eliminates old or damaged blood cells, but the spleen also manufactures the majority of the antibodies that destroy the blood platelets. Since Mary was otherwise medically stable, the removal of the spleen was not an overly serious operation. However, a splenectomy does permanently reduce the body's ability to fight infection and does not fully prevent relapse, although remission of ITP following the operation is 60 to 70 percent.

We talked it over with Mary and her family and agreed that with her platelet count so dangerously low, surgery was the best option.

After the operation, Mary's blood platelet count went up to 333,000, and her purpura and petechiae cleared up. Her prognosis was good, despite the fact that, without a spleen, she suffered from lowered immunity and far greater susceptibility to infection of all kinds.

On a visit to my office eight weeks after her spleen was removed, Mary was satisfied with the results of the operation, but she had a new series of problems to discuss. She complained of constant thirst and the need to urinate frequently. I checked for diabetes and other problems, but she proved to be okay, and the thirst and frequent urination eventually subsided over time. She also suffered from lower back pain and told me that she had tingling feelings and numbness in her legs, feet, and hands. Her neurodermatitis had returned, resulting in infections on her back, arms, and face. She was also still having anxiety-related breathing problems.

In medicine, we often encounter nervous patients like Mary, but a dismissive attitude on the doctor's part can be a barrier to treatment should a serious problem emerge. While stress could explain some of Mary's skin conditions, her petechiae and purpura had been clues to a potentially fatal disease. Although she still had many complaints, Mary was alive to tell the tale and to keep up with her list of medications.

Robert A. Norman is a dermatologist in Tampa, Florida, and the author of The Woman Who Lost Her Skin and Other Dermatological Tales.

CHAPTER

11

A 20-POUND, BONY TUMOR THAT NEARLY SUFFOCATED A MAN FROM THE INSIDE

By W. Roy Smythe

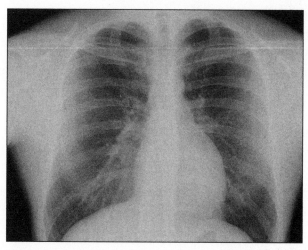

Photo 11-1

One of my junior surgical partners, Scott, called me from the clinic downstairs. "Hey, would you mind coming down?" he asked. "I haven't seen anything like this before." I had never heard Scott so anxious and told him I would be right there.

He met me at the exam room door, wide-eyed, holding the patient's chart in one hand and nervously slapping it into his other palm. "This is wild," he murmured. "A 40-year-old man with bony masses in several areas of his body—hips, face, everywhere. He has one in his chest that we might need to deal with, and soon. This guy is literally suffocating."

We walked over to a computer to take a look at the CT scan.

"Wow, you weren't kidding," I said.

The scan showed a complex bony tumor originating at the ribs and completely filling the left chest. The patient's heart, which would normally rest next to the left lung, was pushed completely against the right lung, compressing it to about half its normal size. And something vital was missing from the scan.

"Where's the left lung?" I asked.

"I don't see it," Scott said.

"Have you had a chance to review his medical history?"

"Not yet," he replied. "I called you as soon as I saw the films."

We opened up the electronic medical record. The patient's name was Hector, and his life had been full of suffering. Since childhood he'd had multiple operations related to these tumors, including removal of his left eye, as well as other craniofacial, hip, and lower-extremity procedures.

Doctors had given him a diagnosis of fibrous dysplasia. This random, or non-inherited, genetic disease involves a mutation in a gene that codes for a protein called Gs, which regulates bone growth. When mutated, the gene causes Gs to go into overdrive, leading to abnormal growth and function of the cells that create bone.

Scott suggested that he and I see the patient together.

We walked down the hall to the clinic exam room and found Hector accompanied by eight women: sisters, cousins, and aunts. My guess was that the average height of the women was at best somewhere around 4-foot-10 and Hector was about 6-foot-7. His head was one and a half times its normal size and severely misshapen. He wore a baseball cap that was about four sizes too small. He had a prosthetic left eye and stood with a stoop, his unusually large hands grasping the handlebar of a walker. He was wearing a nasal cannula—plastic tubing running from an oxygen tank to his nose—and gasped for several seconds each time he spoke.

Polyostotic (literally, "many bones") fibrous dysplasia with endocrine abnormalities is known as McCune-Albright syndrome. While the isolated form of fibrous dysplasia, affecting just one bone or area, occurs in about 20,000 patients in the United States, McCune-Albright affects only 1,000 or so. Hector met the criteria for the syndrome, with diffuse bony masses and acromegaly, an endocrine disorder related to the overproduction of growth hormone, leading to increased height and enlargement of the hands and facial bones.

After introductions, I asked him why he had come to see us now.

"I wanted to know if you could help me," he replied. "I've been fighting this since I was a little boy—first the operations, and then folks making fun of me." He stopped, tears welling up in his eyes. "I can't get around, Doc, and my breathing is really bad." He wiped the tears from his eyes with the back of one of his giant hands. "I want to do normal things, like coach baseball."

"This is going to get worse," I said.

"What are my options, Doc?"

"Removing the mass in your chest is the only chance of getting better," I responded, "but first we need to test your lungs."

When we found that Hector's overall lung function was only about 12 percent of normal, Scott and I met to discuss our next step.

"I don't think he'll survive the surgery," Scott said. "Just removing the bony tumor will not be enough. He needs more lung tissue."

"I know," I said, "but I think we might have a chance."

"How's that?"

"I've operated on patients with bullous disease," I replied, "and this might be similar."

In bullous disease, an area of a patient's lung degenerates from either smoking damage or genetic predisposition, ballooning with air and compressing the adjacent lung tissue over time. When the ballooned area is removed, the normal, compressed lung re-expands.

"This should be the same. Nothing's wrong with his lung; it's just been compressed over time by the mass," I said, trying to sound confident.

"Possibly for decades," Scott added doubtfully. "What if we remove the tumor and there isn't any lung there, or what's there can't re-inflate?"

"Then he won't survive," I conceded. Even though Hector's compromised right lung was functioning, it would not be enough to sustain him through the stress of a major operation, even on a ventilator. He needed both lungs to survive the surgery.

We called Hector and discussed the options. After hearing the risks, he was adamantly against the surgery. But a week later, he changed his mind. "I want to live, but I don't want to live like this," he said. "I'll take my chances, even if they aren't so good."

We typically use a patient's rib cage as a map of sorts. If you open the chest between the third and fourth ribs, for example, you are immediately over the upper heart. If you open between the fifth and sixth, you look right down on the large vessels entering and leaving the lung. Unfortunately, Hector's third through seventh ribs had fused into a huge, solid, bony mass. Rather than opening between the ribs, we had to use surgical saws to work around the entire mass with the goal of lifting it up like the hood of a car.

Once the rib mass was freed from the surrounding tissues, it had to be separated from the center of Hector's chest. This was where the lung would be—if there was any left. The size of a watermelon, the tumor mass was too heavy to lift and hold steady away from the vital organs (heart, esophagus, and possibly the lung). We had to employ a hook and crank system attached to the operating room bed, normally reserved for large orthopedic procedures such as hip replacements, to lift and stabilize the tumor. Then I felt underneath it, where I could not yet see, for the lung. "It's soft tissue," I said, unconvincingly. "But not much of anything there."

"Does it feel like lung?" Scott asked me.

"Not really."

Luckily, the mass had not penetrated the soft tissues, although it had adhered to them as if glued to the surface. We used an electric knife to separate the mass from tissue, then gradually lifted the tumor out of the chest.

Finally it was free. Scott set it on a scale. "Twenty pounds," he said. When he walked back to the table, he saw me staring into the empty space. "Well?" he asked.

At the bottom of the chest cavity was some pink flesh, no more than a tenth of an inch thick. I pointed to the pancake-like tissue. "I think this is the lung," I replied, "but there isn't much."

I looked up at Scott. "Are we going to try to re-inflate it?" he asked.

I turned to the anesthesiologist. No one spoke for several moments. The chest cavity and its thin pink pancake moved gently with the sound of the anesthesia machine—*psssstup, pssssstup*—inflating the right lung.

The breathing tube the anesthesiologist inserts for a lung operation has two channels, one going to each lung. During an operation, one side of the tube is clamped, and the airflow is directed to the lung that isn't being treated. The channel to what we hoped was the left lung was clamped.

"Okay," I said, "unclamp the tube." The machine delivered several breaths. . . . Nothing.

Suddenly, a couple of small areas popped up, like pink bubblegum bubbles, on the pink tissue. Then a few more. The pancake thickened, and thickened again, and then more bubbles grew and coalesced with others. In three minutes the entire lung had re-inflated from a flat, spongy nothing to a complete lung 30 times larger. "It's working," the anesthesiologist reported. "Good oxygen exchange from that lung!"

"Impossible," Scott murmured under his breath. "Impossible."

Within a month, Hector was off oxygen and getting around without a walker. Not long after, I caught a glimpse of him on a local television news spot. I was across the room and the television volume was low, but I saw him smiling, surrounded by little boys in baseball caps.

W. Roy Smythe is chairman of surgery for the Texas A&M Health Science Center College of Medicine.

CHAPTER

12

FAR FROM OKAY

By W. Roy Smythe

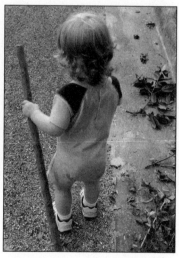

Photo 12-1

I was reviewing my emails late in the day when I found a message flagged "Important" in the subject line. It was from Kelsey, one of our hospital's new pediatric surgeons. "Consulted regarding a 16-month-old with a middle mediastinal mass," her message read. "Compression of trachea. Would love your thoughts."

The mass Kelsey referred to in her email was in an area where a lot of things can go wrong. It's what we call the mediastinum—the middle of the chest between the lungs where several important organs, such as the heart, trachea, and esophagus, reside.

As a thoracic surgeon, I specialize in operating on organs in this area and often review cases with colleagues.

I responded that I'd be happy to speak with her, and in less than 15 minutes she was tapping on my door. Kelsey was obviously very concerned about this one, so I quickly pulled the CT scan of the mass up on the computer as she relayed the details of the case. The patient was a 16-month-old boy who was developing normally but had recently been diagnosed with asthma.

He had been admitted to the hospital because of increasing stridor, a high-pitched sound made during inhalation. Stridor indicates a narrowing somewhere in the main, or proximal, airways—the area of the respiratory tract between the vocal cords high in the neck and where the trachea, or windpipe, branches to meet the two lungs. Stridor is often thought to indicate asthma, but it usually doesn't. Asthmatics make a different sound: a wheeze. Wheezes occur during exhalation and imply obstruction of the smaller airways that are in the lungs themselves.

The boy's name was Ian, and it was clear that his breathing problems were not caused by asthma. The CT images showed a 5-centimeter mass—about the size of a lemon—narrowing his trachea by more than half and encasing the adjacent esophagus, which carries food from the mouth to the stomach. It looked as if malevolent bees had built a rounded, ill-formed hive in Ian's chest.

I took in a deep breath. "That looks bad, Kelsey."

"Yeah," she replied. "It may be malignant. I'm worried about a sarcoma."

We knew that about half of mediastinal tumors in children are malignant—aggressive cancers that grow into surrounding organs. Such tumors can take various forms. Sarcomas are malignant tumors of connective tissues such as muscle and bone. Tumors can also form in the lymph glands, the small organs of the immune system that filter bacteria from the bloodstream. Mediastinal tumors are rare, however. A total of 10,000 children are diagnosed with cancer every year in the United States, and mediastinal tumors account for about 100 of those cases.

"If not a tumor, I guess this could be a fistula," Kelsey said, "with a chicken bone or something lodged there and causing an infection."

A fistula is an abnormal connection of tissue between two organs. There are a group of congenital fistulas that can connect the trachea and esophagus, which grow from the same embryonic tissue. If a child swallows an object that lodges in the fistula, it can trigger an infection that may result in an inflamed mass. But Kelsey said that Ian's white blood cell count and other tests that would indicate an infection were normal.

I considered whether we should get other tests, such as a biopsy or an MRI. "We could," Kelsey replied. "But if the mass enlarges, it will block the trachea completely. I think we just have to go for it."

We discussed the challenges of removing Ian's mass surgically. If it was attached to the esophagus extensively, we would have to remove much of the organ and replace it with a section of the stomach. The tracheal part of the procedure could get even more complex. The trachea does not heal as reliably as the esophagus, and only a small amount of tissue can be removed from it for reconstruction, giving us a narrower margin of error in the event of damage and subsequent repair. The complexities and risks were so great that Kelsey and I sought the input of other doctors as well. Kelsey called her mentor at the pediatric surgical program where she had trained, and I called a pediatric surgeon who had trained with me years earlier. These colleagues felt surgery was unavoidable.

We scheduled Ian's operation and went to see him and his family in the pediatric ward. While we talked, Ian stood in his crib, sucking his pacifier.

We did our best to assuage the parents' fears, but this was a lot of surgery for a little person, and it involved a great deal of risk. Whether or not we found a malignancy, the outcome might be bad.

After a night of little sleep for me, and most likely less for Ian's parents, the morning of the surgery arrived. In the operating room, nurses carefully inserted a breathing tube into Ian's narrowed airway. He was then anesthetized, positioned with his right side up, and cleaned with an antiseptic solution. Drapes covered his tiny body, exposing only the operative field.

We made an incision in his chest and placed retractors to make room between his ribs. The mass was immediately evident. It was oval-shaped, with an irregular contour, like the surface of a reddish-tan rock. We both felt it. "It's fixed and firm," said Kelsey, not needing to mention that this was consistent with a cancerous tumor. We began by working our way around the mass with surgical scissors to the back wall of the esophagus. It was a struggle.

"It's definitely involving the esophagus," I said. "Let's try the trachea." Kelsey was a skilled young surgeon, but using a variety of tools, including an electric scalpel, we could not free the mass from either structure. It was too firmly attached. While working around the mass, we spotted an enlarged lymph node nearby. "That's not a good sign," I murmured. "Might have spread there."

We worked without speaking—four adult hands in a small space. A sense of foreboding was accumulating in the room around us like fog.

Finally, I made a desperate suggestion. "Let's divide the mass," I said. "Maybe we can see from another perspective how it's attached to the trachea and esophagus separately—we aren't making progress."

This was something we preferred not to do. When removing a tumor, an "en masse" approach is best, meaning the entire tumor is extracted intact with any surrounding tissues attached, which gives surgeons the best chance to leave no cancerous tissue behind.

"Agreed," Kelsey replied. "Maybe we can save some of the trachea that way, make the repair easier."

I took a scalpel and carefully incised the mass. After a couple of passes, it cracked open. Ian's heartbeat, a beep on the anesthesia monitor, registered five times before either of us spoke.

There was something dark and linear at the center. It looked horrifyingly like a slug.

"What is that?" Kelsey asked.

I reached down and grasped it with a pair of forceps. "It's firm," I said. Kelsey adjusted the light overhead—there was a glint of reflection. "Metal?" I asked. I carefully pulled the object free. It was dark gray, oval, and covered in a layer of mucus.

I held it up in the light between us.

It was a leaf.

"A leaf?" Kelsey asked. "A leaf?" Her eyes were squinting above her mask, and her forehead wrinkled in disbelief. Suddenly it was clear. The mass formed to protect Ian's body from the leaf and had taken on a life of its own. We both started laughing. The nurses clapped. There was no cancer; Ian was going to survive.

During the rest of the operation, we found that the leaf was nestled in a place where the normally cylindrical esophageal wall bulged out—a diverticulum in medical jargon. It all added up. Ian had swallowed an oak leaf months before, and it had lodged in the diverticulum, unable to pass. The leaf's tip had eroded into the trachea and eventually, after white blood cells honed in on the region to heal the lesion, a scar formed around both the inflamed tissue and the leaf.

The young mother and father were incredibly relieved at the news, which Kelsey and I delivered immediately following the operation. They hugged each other, and after several moments, Kelsey and I left the room quietly, the two of them still embracing. Ian left the hospital after a few days. He was going to be fine.

The fact that the mass was not a malignant tumor didn't change the urgency behind the operation. If Ian's diagnosis of stridor and the surgery had been delayed, the mass could have led to the complete obstruction of the airway and sudden suffocation, or a leakage of esophageal contents, laden with bacteria from the mouth. If leaked into the trachea, these contents could have led to pneumonia, or if into the mediastinum, to sepsis and vascular collapse. We were relieved to find that the mass was not cancer, but left untreated, a simple leaf could very well have ended Ian's life.

W. Roy Smythe is chairman of surgery for the Texas A&M Health Science Center College of Medicine.

CHAPTER

13

SAVE THE LINEBACKER

By W. Roy Smythe

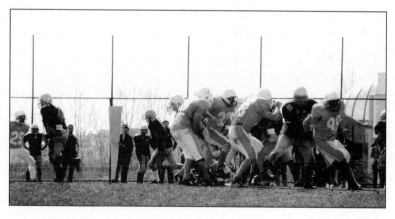

Photo 13-1

College football has 8,000 injuries a year, but that's not the only reason players visit the ER.

Early in my career, I was the resident on call one night in the cardiothoracic intensive care unit when an emergency room doctor called and asked me to come down and see a patient. "Young guy," he said. "He has some sort of an airway problem."

Those were worrisome words, because airway problems can be immediately life-threatening. I rushed to the patient's examining room, where two men were supporting a third, younger man. One of the two supporting him was grasping his upper arm so tightly that his own arms were visibly shaking. He looked very scared.

"I'm Steve's dad, Doc." He looked at the man on the other side of the patient. "And this is Coach Alexander."

"Hey, Doc," grunted the coach. "Somethin' ain't right here. This is one tough kid."

I walked around to the other side of the bed so I could see the patient. Steve was about 20. His forearms, biceps, and triceps, under stress as he leaned forward on the bed, were well developed and defined. His hands were large, with abrasions on his knuckles. He was wearing a white and blue athletic shirt and a matching cap with the logo of a local college. He was sweating, despite the fact that it was cool in the ER. He was extremely short of breath, and his shoulder and upper-back muscles, evidently called into play to supplement the usual ones, were heaving in concert with the movements of his chest.

"Steve, what's up?" I asked.

He replied without looking up at me, gasping between words. "I felt a little . . . weird . . . the last couple of days . . . and then got . . . a cold or something . . . really . . . hard to breathe . . . now."

"What happened to your knuckles?" I asked.

He looked up, managing a crooked grin on his red, sweaty face, and replied, "Linebacker."

At that moment, the emergency room resident walked in. "We have the CT scan," he said.

A BASIC PROCEDURE GOES AWRY

We walked over and looked at the scan on a monitor. I was stunned. There was a huge mass, the size and shape of a small cantaloupe, in Steve's upper chest. It was compressing the area where the trachea splits into two smaller tubes, called the main-stem bronchi. The right main-stem bronchus was obliterated, and the left was only about half its normal diameter.

"This explains why he wants to lean forward," I said. "It takes pressure off his airway."

"What do you think it is?" the emergency room resident asked.

"I don't know," I said, "but a lymphoma has to be high on the list." A tumor originating from the white blood cells of the immune system, lymphoma represents almost 15 percent of all cancer diagnoses in young adults. Steve's symptoms had come on quickly, and of the tumors that can occur in this area of the chest, lymphoma is one of the fastest.

We took Steve to the operating room to biopsy the mass. The staff surgeon asked me to have the anesthesiologist insert the breathing tube into the patient's airway while he was awake and sitting upright. Although patients are usually sedated and paralyzed during this procedure, the surgeon worried that if Steve were relaxed and lying down, the tumor could press on the airway so firmly that the anesthesiologist would be unable to pass the breathing tube at all—what we term "losing the airway."

As I walked into the OR, the anesthesiologist was lowering Steve from a sitting to a lying position, counter to the surgeon's instructions.

"We think you should intubate him awake and upright," I said hurriedly, "due to the tumor's location."

"I don't think that is necessary," he replied, and immediately injected Steve with the intravenous anesthetic.

Over the next several seconds, I watched in horror as the anesthesiologist tried five times to pass the tube, only to have it stop halfway down: the tumor had slammed the trachea shut.

"Dammit!" the anesthesiologist said, "it won't go!" His face was red, and his hands trembled from anxiety.

I ran over to the bedside and barked at the circulating nurse, "Get the rigid bronchoscope, stat!"

Unlike the thinner and flexible breathing tube, the rigid bronchoscope is not much more than a metal tube about half an inch in diameter with a lighted fiber optic shaft. We occasionally use this device to remove foreign bodies or to biopsy airway tumors. It can also be used to ventilate a patient when the more flexible breathing tube cannot be inserted.

As the nurse ran out of the room, I looked over at Steve's oxygen saturation monitor, which displays the amount of oxygen being carried by the red blood cells to the tissues of the body. The monitor both displays a number and beeps with each heartbeat; the beeping tone gets lower as the numbers go down.

A normal blood saturation level is between 95 and 100 percent. Anything lower than 80 percent for more than a few minutes can damage the brain and other organs and possibly result in death. With no oxygen reaching Steve's lungs, I listened and watched helplessly as the numbers got smaller and the beeping tone went lower: 90 . . . 70 . . . 52 . . . Steve's heartbeat began to slow and became irregular.

"We're losing him!" I yelled. I knew that CPR would be futile—it pushes oxygen through the airway, and the airway was closed.

The nurse wheeled a cart into the room. I grabbed a rigid bronchoscope and attached the light cord as the anesthesiologist moved out of the way. I placed the scope in Steve's mouth, identified the larynx, and shoved the metal scope past the vocal cords. I felt a bump as it slid past the tumor and down the left main-stem bronchus. I heaved a sigh of relief. We could deliver enough oxygen to one side to sustain him. Now I just needed tubing to hook the bronchoscope to the ventilator.

"Hand me the ventilator tubing," I told the anesthesiologist.

"Thank God!" he said, handing me the tubing.

I froze. The tubing, retrieved in haste by the nurse, was the wrong size and lacked the connective hardware the device required. "Get me a connector!" I yelled. The nurse ran out of the room again.

A DESPERATE GAMBIT

All of the alarms on the machine were now going off. Steve's oxygen saturation was 25 percent, and his heartbeat was erratic.

We were out of time and had to do something immediately or Steve was going to suffocate right in front of us. I suddenly flashed back to the way I had been taught as a medical student to do mouth-to-mouth resuscitation, and it triggered an idea. Desperate, I began to blow into the tube—something that isn't part of any standard medical procedure.

"What the hell are you doing?" the anesthesiologist shouted. But within seconds the saturation was up to 50, then 65, then the low 80s. Steve's heartbeat normalized.

The air we exhale has lower oxygen content than what we normally breathe in, but it is close, and much better than nothing.

I was acting like a human ventilator, delivering enough oxygen to sustain Steve's life.

As the operating staff looked on, dumbfounded, I continued breathing through the tube. Eventually the nurse found a fitting, and we hooked Steve to a proper ventilator, from which 100 percent oxygen could be delivered. I was finally able to make an incision above his breastbone and biopsy the tumor. We sent a piece of the mass to the pathology lab down the hall. A few minutes later the pathologist called. It was probable lymphoma.

The best treatment for lymphoma in the airway is chemotherapy, not surgery, so we called in an oncologist who was able to administer chemotherapy in the operating room. We then transferred Steve to the ICU with the rigid scope still in his airway. The plan was to try to shrink the tumor with the tube in place, protecting his airway from collapsing again.

The pathologic examination showed that Steve's cancer was related to acute lymphoblastic leukemia, which can spread very rapidly. But the prognosis in young adults is much better than in older age groups. Some 75 percent of cases in young patients are curable.

Steve underwent more chemotherapy while still on the ventilator. Luckily, despite the size and dangerous location of his tumor, Steve was a fighter and was soon breathing on his own. The tumor shrank, and he got more good news when we found the cancer had not spread to his bone marrow. On his tenth day in the hospital, he was transferred out of intensive care.

A week later, as I was walking across the hospital lobby, I encountered a gratifying sight: two men supporting a third as they walked toward the front door. Steve's father and coach were taking him home.

W. Roy Smythe is chairman of surgery for the Texas A&M Health Science Center College of Medicine.

CHAPTER

14

"WE CAN TAKE HIS HEART OUT, REMOVE THE TUMOR, AND PUT IT BACK IN"

By W. Roy Smythe

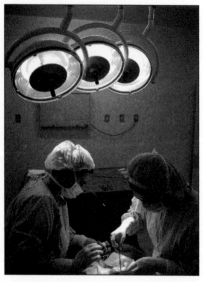

Photo 14-1

I was in the middle of a normal clinic day, seeing candidates for surgery, when a nurse told me that one of them had arrived with a diagnostic video. When I had a free moment, I walked over to a computer and put the CD into the drive. As the program booted up, I noticed that the video was a cardiac MRI study. I clicked through the images, and what I saw was frightening. A large mass was growing in the patient's heart, in the back wall of the left atrial chamber, one of the worst possible places to have a problem like this. The right atrium and both ventricles are somewhat accessible to the surgeon's knife. But the left atrium at the back of the heart next to the spine is a difficult, if not impossible, area to reach.

As I watched the video, more details emerged. As the left atrium attempted to pump blood, the wall opposite the growth ballooned out awkwardly instead of contracting with the rest of the chamber, its movement altered by the growth. The mass also took up a lot of space and was impeding blood flow. If it got just 5 percent larger, the chamber would be almost completely obstructed, resulting in a high risk of sudden death.

I called one of my cardiac surgery colleagues, Mike Reardon, and asked him to take a look.

"Oh, man," Mike said, "that's a tumor, all right—and in a bad place."

My own heart sank. Primary tumors, which originate in tissues rather than spreading there from some other place in the body, are uncommon in the heart. They occur in less than 0.05 percent of autopsies. Seventy-five percent of them are benign, but this one did not look harmless. Benign tumors typically grow out from the surface of the cardiac wall like a mushroom on a stalk; malignant tumors look more like a bulge of varying thickness in the wall.

Most cardiac surgeons will encounter only a few benign primary tumors in a career, and many will never deal with a malignant one.

"If we were to think about removing it," I asked, "how would we approach it?"

"How old is the patient?"

"Thirty-seven," I answered.

"Any history of coronary disease?"

"The transfer notes don't mention anything."

"Good," said Mike. "There might be one way to remove this, but it is drastic. We can take his heart out of his body, remove the tumor, reconstruct the heart, and put it back in."

"Okay . . . wow," was all I could say.

He was describing an extremely rare procedure: a cardiac auto-transplant. We would operate on the heart outside the chest cavity and use cardiopulmonary bypass to support his body while we worked. The first successful auto-transplant to remove a cardiac tumor was performed in the 1990s. Since then, the procedure has been undertaken fewer than 50 times worldwide.

Mike and I went into the exam room to discuss the options with the patient, Mr. Johnson, and his wife. We told him the mass was probably a cardiac sarcoma, a malignant tumor originating in either the heart muscle or the blood vessels located there. We also told him that he faced significant risk of sudden death if the chamber became completely blocked, and that chemotherapy was usually ineffective for larger tumors of this type. Surgery was the only reasonable option, and we needed to move fast.

"However," I said, "there will be a fair amount of risk."

"How much risk?" Mr. Johnson asked quickly.

"There are three things to worry about," I replied. "One is whether or not we can remove the entire tumor. The second is whether we can put the heart back together again so it will function normally. And the last thing is the overall risk of having to stop your heart, remove it, fix it, put it back in, and restart it.

"We normally quote a 1 to 5 percent risk of dying for heart surgery," I continued, "but your risk will be higher. The best-case scenario, if all goes well, is perhaps a 10 percent risk, and the worst case would be maybe five times that."

There was no hesitation. "Let's do this," Mr. Johnson said.

Two days later we were in the operating room, where I would assist Mike. As the anesthetizing medications were administered, Mr. Johnson's blood pressure dropped dangerously. The anesthesia team quickly gave him epinephrine to bring it back up. "Not much blood getting into that left side," the anesthesiologist said as he looked at the monitor. "That's why his pressure dropped. Good thing you didn't wait too much longer."

We divided Johnson's sternum and placed retractors to open up the chest. We then cut into the pericardium, the outer sac protecting the heart, and inserted tubing into the large vessels entering and leaving the heart to allow blood to bypass the organ.

"Go on bypass," Mike said, loudly enough for the technicians managing the pump behind us to hear. The heart began to empty of blood.

We put a cold saline slush around the organ to help put it into a kind of suspended animation. Then Mike and I went to work, using surgical scissors and scalpels to sever the vessels entering and leaving the heart. Once the large vessels and other attachments were cut, Mike lifted the organ out of the body.

I looked into Mr. Johnson's open chest as Mike placed this cold, now flaccid heart on an operating table a few feet away. Where his heart should have been was a void with tubes leaving it from the margins.

The only other time a doctor has this view is during a heart transplant, after the removal of the diseased organ and immediately before placing a donor heart into the recipient's chest. The difference in this situation, however, was critical. During a transplant, we never take out the diseased heart until we have the new one in the room. In this case, there was no new heart and a chance we wouldn't be able to fix the one we had taken out.

Mike and I worked quickly at the table, using our scalpels to remove the tumor.

"It's bigger than it looked in the images," Mike said, "but I think we got all of it."

We placed the tumor and the portion of the fleshy heart wall that we removed in a small plastic bucket to transfer to a pathologist. He would check the tissue to make sure that we had removed the entire mass.

A few moments later, the pathologist called into the room. "There is some microscopic tumor at the margin," he said.

Mike stared down at the opening in the back of the heart where the tumor had been.

"If we take any more," he said, "we may not be able to reconstruct it."

"We can try chemotherapy," I replied. "It has a better chance of working with microscopic disease. Better to have a chance than not to leave the OR."

"I agree," he said. "We don't have much time. We need to get this organ back in there."

He sewed a piece of bovine pericardium—the heart sac from a cow—into the opening left by the removed tumor. We then carried the heart back over to the patient and placed it in the void.

We sewed the large vessels back together and allowed the heart to gradually warm. We knew that a healthy organ will often start to beat once it is warmed, even without a blood supply reestablished.

But nothing happened.

We continued to work, completing the suture lines. Blood began to flow back into the coronary vessels.

"No action here," the anesthesiologist said, watching the electrocardiogram.

Mike inserted a small needle into the muscle to measure the temperature. "Should be working; the temp is good," he said.

Several more seconds passed. Still nothing.

Then we noticed a quiver near the apex of the heart, followed by another, and then the heart sprang back to life, beating vigorously. We removed the tubes and closed Mr. Johnson's sternum.

Our patient made a good recovery and was discharged from the hospital several days later. After a regimen of chemotherapy to treat the microscopic tumor left on the heart, he had a good chance of complete remission and possibly even a cure.

W. Roy Smythe is chairman of surgery for the Texas A&M Health Science Center College of Medicine.

CHAPTER

15

AN UNWELCOME RINGING

By Christopher Linstrom

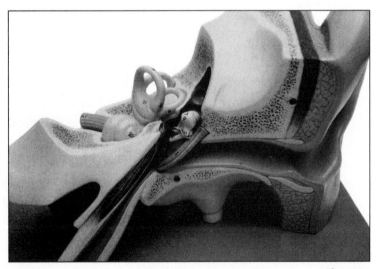

Photo 15-1

By the time Stephen came to my office complaining of painful
spasms and ringing in both ears, he had already been to
several physicians about his problem. He had been given an array

of diagnoses; most doctors said he had acute outer or middle ear infections and prescribed oral antibiotics or ear drops. These measures had not helped, though. He was 21 years old and had suffered with this pain for nearly a year.

Like many people with ear or head sounds—which we lump into one word, tinnitus—Stephen was distraught. Knowing that there is no magic drug for ringing, I mentally prepared my usual sermonette: avoid noise, aspirin, and methylxanthines (stimulants of the central nervous system, such as caffeine). And embrace the tried-and-true helper, sound substitution, or "masking." This technique, in my experience, is a remedy for almost every patient with tinnitus.

Then Stephen delivered the bombshell. "I've been treated twice with extended courses of intravenous antibiotics for Lyme disease," he told me. "In fact, I have an intravenous line in my arm right now and am just finishing an eight-week course of Rocephin [an antibiotic] for my second bout of Lyme. I've had to drop out of college because the pulses in my ears are so bad I can't concentrate on anything. Could it be related to Lyme?" The spasms were occurring every few seconds in both of his ears throughout his entire waking day, he continued. The associated pain was so severe that his whole life revolved around dealing with it. Clearly this was not the typical case of tinnitus.

Stephen was first exposed to Lyme disease, a tick-borne infection, as a child while playing in the woods near his home in Westchester County, New York. He was re-infected as a college student in 2007. Severe cases of Lyme disease can involve cardiac or neurological symptoms and are often treated with the intravenous antibiotic ceftriaxone. But I was unaware of any link between Lyme disease and pulsatile tinnitus. Otherwise,

Stephen was in stable health with no other contributory medical or surgical problems.

I examined his right ear with a microscope and an ear speculum. There it was, apparent right away in an otherwise normal eardrum: the drum pulsed and appeared to go into spasms in an irregular way. I observed the exact same thing in the left ear. There was no mass behind either drum, and the middle ear clefts on each side were normal. My exam did find spasms of his soft palate (palatal myoclonus) and twitching around his eyes (blepharospasm), but these were not as bothersome to him as the pulsing. I had never before seen a patient like this.

It was time to put Stephen through some proper hearing tests to find out what was going on. The middle ear has two muscles, the tensor tympani and the stapedius. The stapedius and, to a lesser extent, the tensor tympani engage in the acoustic reflex (or the middle ear muscle reflex), a contraction in response to loud sounds. A reflex is an involuntary motor response, so it is present both while a person is awake and while unconscious. All reflexes follow a looping nerve response: an arc toward the central nervous system, called the afferent limb, and an arc away from the central nervous system to the end organ, termed the efferent limb. For the middle ear muscle reflex, the afferent limb is the auditory nerve; the efferent limb is the facial nerve for the stapedius muscle and the trigeminal nerve for the tensor tympani muscle. The reflex itself occurs in the brain stem, one of the deepest and most basic parts of the brain.

The stapedius responds by tightening the mobility of the stapes (or "stirrup"), and the tensor tympani tightens the eardrum and pulls the malleus ("hammer"). The stapes and malleus are tiny bones that transmit hearing through the inner ear. By restricting the motion of the stapes, the stapedius may be able to dampen loud sounds coming toward the ear, but that response does not happen quickly enough to prevent acoustic trauma from fast-acting sounds, such as a gun blast. The acoustic reflex is also thought to play a role in preventing us from hearing our own voices as we speak. Although we know that the reflex is present in healthy individuals and we evaluate it as part of every complete hearing test, its ultimate function is not entirely understood.

To investigate Stephen's ear spasms, I ordered a complete hearing test. Any neurological process involving two or more cranial nerves almost always points the finger of diagnostic suspicion to the brain stem, which is the anatomical takeoff point of the cranial nerves. So I also ordered an MRI of my patient's brain, with and without contrast enhancement, to get a good look at that area.

The tests showed that Stephen's hearing was completely normal, but the acoustic reflexes could not be tested because of the ongoing spasms in each ear. The MRI of his brain was entirely normal as well. At this point, my most likely diagnosis was myoclonus (muscle spasm) of either or both the stapedius and tensor tympani muscles. The painful eardrum spasms were the result of the contractions of one or both of the middle ear muscles.

All physicians are trained to begin by thinking broadly and then apply reasonable medical and surgical measures to the most likely cause of the clinical problem. Physicians are also trained to treat medically first and to reserve surgery for cases that fail medical management. Because Stephen had already been treated for Lyme with intravenous antibiotics, I suggested a consultation with a neurologist and perhaps a short trial of common medications used for either seizure or peripheral neuropathy, such as Tegretol or gabapentin. Tegretol decreases the spread of seizure; it is also used to treat bipolar disorder and trigeminal neuralgia, a condition causing severe facial pain. Gabapentin is a molecule related to gamma-aminobutyric acid, or GABA, a common neurotransmitter. It has well-studied analgesic and anticonvulsant effects, although its exact mechanism of action is unknown. Gabapentin is used for a variety of neurological disorders, including spasm and extremity pain.

Stephen began with a short course of Tegretol, prescribed by his neurologist. It did not lessen the symptoms or block the spasms, so I started Stephen on gabapentin. After a few weeks, he reported that it had no beneficial effect either.

Understandably anxious, Stephen had sought a few other consultations, with conflicting recommendations. I suggested he see a colleague of mine in Boston who had a great deal of experience with Eustachian tube dysfunction. The Boston doctor made a small opening in Stephen's left eardrum and inserted a microscopic telescope attached to a video camera to visualize the middle ear muscles. All of this was done under topical anesthesia while Stephen was awake. The results matched my diagnosis but added an important new piece of information: The offending muscle was the tensor tympani muscle, not the stapedius.

Now that we had identified the culprit, how to treat it? There were two possibilities: injecting a neuromuscular-blocking medication, such as botulinum toxin (Botox), into the tensor tympani muscle in the middle ear, or cutting the muscle surgically. The former would be a temporary trial that would wear off in about 6 to 12 weeks. The second option would be permanent. There were potential risks associated with either choice. First, either temporarily or permanently blocking the muscle might not solve the problem. Second, loud sounds coming toward the treated ear might seem even louder than before. Stephen considered his options and, after speaking with his parents, decided to have the muscle cut. He had been suffering with the spasms for so long that he did not want to try a temporary solution.

I started with the left ear because it was the more bothersome. The surgery was all done through the outer ear channel; it involved making small incisions around the eardrum so it could be turned aside like the page of a book. The eardrum was then dissected off the hammer bone to allow me to see the tensor tympani muscle as it approaches the hammer bone at its narrow neck. The nerve to Stephen's face runs in a bony channel near the tensor tympani muscle. We monitored his face with an electromyography system, which allowed me to electrically stimulate the facial nerve and make sure it was not being injured by the surgery. I then found and divided the tensor tympani muscle, first partially with a small knife and then completely with a scalpel-like laser. I placed a small amount of packing under the eardrum, turned it back into its usual place, put some packing material over the eardrum, and bandaged the ear. Stephen was awakened and transferred to the recovery room.

About an hour later, my patient was fully awake and ready to go home. I went to see him in the patient recovery area and he exclaimed, "It's gone! I think it's really gone!" His parents were as overjoyed as he was. It appeared that his long nightmare might finally be ending. Fast-forward several weeks: the surgery did in fact abolish the spasm in Stephen's left ear. His hearing remained normal, and the spasms around his left eye subsided.

About six weeks after the left side, I operated on the right ear in a similar fashion. This side also healed, and the spasms went away with no significant side effects. Today Stephen has resumed his university studies and is getting his life back on track.

I still had not addressed Stephen's original question: was Lyme disease responsible for his ear agonies? I would say yes. The disease certainly has many far-reaching neurological symptoms. As Sir William Osler, regarded by many as the father of modern medicine, said many years ago, "He who knows syphilis knows medicine." Of course, syphilis was not Stephen's problem, but the cause of Lyme disease, Borrelia burgdorferi, is in the same family as the causative agent of syphilis, Treponema pallidum. They are both spirochetes, bacteria that cause an insidious range of health issues.

For me, Stephen's case reinforced the notion that the medical history, as detailed by the patient himself or herself, is the most important part of any medical or surgical encounter. Patients who have difficult medical conditions are usually good historians: They live with the problem all day, every day, and can reflect upon its origins and its clinical course. The patient almost always provides all of the diagnostic clues to the solution, guiding the physician in where to look and how to treat.

Christopher Linstrom is an otologist/neurotologist and professor of otolaryngology at the New York Eye and Ear Infirmary.

CHAPTER
16

MISDIAGNOSING ADHD

By Mark Cohen

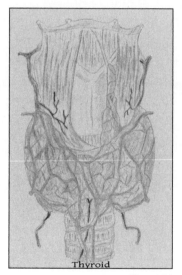

Photo 16-1

I was at my desk dictating a report when one of our pediatric endocrinologists knocked on my open door.

"Hi, Mark," she said. "I have a 12-year-old patient whose mother is worried that she may have ADHD [attention deficit hyperactivity disorder]. She says her daughter has been getting more and more inattentive and disorganized and takes a long time to finish her homework. Her lab tests show that she might have resistance to thyroid hormone, which I know can cause ADHD symptoms. I'm not convinced she has that—because it's pretty rare—but I'm also not sure she has ADHD. Since you know more about ADHD than I do, I'd like to get your opinion."

"I'll be happy to take a look. I'll let you know what I think after I see her."

The young lady and her mother showed up about a week later, bringing a folder of report cards bearing A's and B's.

"How long have you been concerned about her?" I asked her mother.

"For about the past year or so she's been having difficulty in school," she replied. "She does her work, but then forgets to turn it in. She tells me it sometimes takes her four hours to do an hour's worth of homework."

These are common complaints regarding children with ADHD. ADHD is a chronic condition that causes inattention and difficulty in organizing. Most children with ADHD also show impulsivity and hyperactive behavior, but a sizable number have problems only with attention and focusing. The term ADHD is now used for the hyperactive and non-hyperactive forms of this disorder.

There is no specific laboratory test for ADHD. It is diagnosed by determining if a child has a significant number of inattentive, hyperactive, and impulsive symptoms; if they are excessive for the child's age; if they have been present since early childhood and in more than one setting; and if they cannot be explained by some other physical, mental, or emotional condition. So I asked the girl's mother questions designed to detect the symptoms of ADHD.

Her responses showed no hints of impulsivity or hyperactivity. That in itself wasn't a surprise. Children, especially girls, with the inattentive form of ADHD are often not diagnosed until middle school because of their lack of disruptive behavior. But as I continued questioning, it became clear that this patient did not have ADHD at all. Not only had her symptoms all started within the past year but she did not have enough of the ADHD symptoms to merit the diagnosis. Something else was going on.

Her chart noted that about six months previously her mother had brought up her daughter's picky appetite and slow growth. Because there was a family history of thyroid problems, the pediatrician had ordered basic blood tests of thyroid function, although she expected they would be normal. In fact, they were not—an important clue.

The thyroid gland, a small butterfly-shaped structure situated low in the front of the neck, controls the growth and metabolism of almost every organ in the body. It produces two related hormones, called T4 (or thyroxine) and T3 (or triiodothyronine). The release of these hormones is triggered by the pituitary gland, which secretes a substance called TSH (thyroid-stimulating hormone) that regulates thyroid production in a feedback loop. In hypothyroidism, the supply of thyroid hormones does not keep up with the body's demands, and the TSH level is high, reflecting the body's need to prod for more thyroid production. In hyperthyroidism, when the thyroid gland is producing too much of its hormones, the TSH level drops to zero.

In nearly half the cases of hyperthyroidism in youths, the cause is an autoimmune condition known as Graves' disease. (The other half is caused by growths on the thyroid.) For some unknown reason, in Graves' disease, the body begins to produce antibodies against the thyroid gland, which causes the gland to enlarge and produce more thyroid hormones. Typically, someone with this condition will have symptoms of hyperthyroidism, which can include fatigue, heat intolerance, sweating, palpitations (the physical awareness of a rapid heart rate), and weight loss.

What had puzzled the endocrinologist about our patient was that her thyroid hormone levels were high, but her TSH was normal. This pattern is seen in the syndrome of resistance to thyroid hormone, a rare condition in which the body is insensitive to cues regulating the thyroid hormone feedback loop. I went back and reviewed the literature on ADHD and thyroid hormone resistance. When thyroid hormone resistance was first described in 1967, doctors noticed that the children had enlarged thyroids. Later on, doctors noticed that the children sometimes seemed hyperactive and nervous, resembling children with ADHD. For a time, checking the thyroid function of children with a diagnosis of ADHD was sometimes done. Eventually, doctors noticed that children with thyroid hormone resistance were more prone to learning disabilities than children with ADHD. Some were also inattentive and hyperactive.

This adolescent girl's picture was becoming even more confusing. She had symptoms that looked like ADHD, but she clearly did not have ADHD. She had a high thyroid hormone level that looked like Graves' disease, but didn't have the low TSH level that went with it. Although her blood tests suggested that her body's thyroid-TSH feedback system wasn't working properly, she didn't display the ADHD-like symptoms of hyperactivity and nervousness that are typical of thyroid hormone resistance.

After the girl and her mother left, I walked down the hall to the endocrinologist's office. "Well, she doesn't have ADHD," I said. "And she doesn't have the typical hyperactive symptoms that are described with thyroid hormone resistance. So I'm stumped."

She smiled. "I was hoping you'd say that," she said. "I don't think she has thyroid hormone resistance. She's got plain old Graves' disease. She's just hyperthyroid."

"But what about the TSH?" I asked. "Shouldn't that be low in Graves' disease?"

"Yes, and that's the tricky part. I was suspicious, because her symptoms didn't fit the lab results, so I sent her blood to an academic lab in Chicago. They told me her TSH is actually very low. It turns out that she has an unusual antibody that reacts with the standard TSH test and gives a falsely high reading."

"Okay, but how does hyperthyroidism fit with her symptoms? I still can't explain why she is so inattentive and disorganized."

The endocrinologist then told me that in children and adolescents, the earliest indications of hyperthyroidism may be behavioral, like hyperactivity, nervousness, or moodiness. Forgetfulness and inattention—just like our patient's symptoms—are common. That was something I hadn't known, never having had a patient with early Graves' disease, but it certainly made sense.

We started our patient on methimazole, a medication that decreases the production of thyroid hormone. Within a few months, she was back to earning straight A's and finishing her homework in nothing flat. Her mother was thrilled. So was I.

Mark Cohen is a pediatrician in Santa Clara, California.

CHAPTER

17

A SWOLLEN AREA GROWS
LARGER AND LARGER

By Mark Cohen

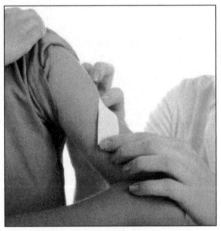

Photo 17-1

My second-year resident ducked his head into my office in the pediatric clinic. "Hey, Dr. Cohen," he said, "can you come and look at a girl with a lump on her arm?"

The area on the 7-year-old girl's upper right arm had been swelling for about a week, he said, and it was getting bigger. She'd had a slight fever about a week ago, but none since. The lump was painful and hard, and yesterday the mother had noticed some slight redness of the skin. The child had been healthy, and her immunizations were up to date. She wasn't taking any medications, and no one at home had been ill. The resident noted that she hadn't had any injury, such as a bite, or any exposure to animals.

We went in to see the girl. I introduced myself and crouched down beside her.

"Hi. Can I check your arm?"

She held out her arm, a wary look on her face. I began by examining her wrist and forearm, carefully feeling the tissue.

Kids' lumps and bumps are usually benign. But sometimes they prove to be diagnostic challenges, and every once in a while they turn out to be a sign of something very serious. When a child comes in with a lump, the remote but real possibility of a tumor is always in the back of my mind. A malignant tumor often feels rock hard, as opposed to an enlarged lymph node, which is usually firm but not hard, or a cyst, which might feel soft.

"Does that hurt?" I asked. She shook her head. "Good. Can you show me where the bump is?" She pointed to the inside of her upper arm. I could see the swelling, right where the bicep muscle makes contact with the bone. My fingers slid lightly over the surface of the faintly reddened spot, then probed a little deeper. The child winced a bit, but she did not seem to be in great pain.

The swollen area was about the size of a matchbook. It felt too hard to be a benign enlarged lymph node, and it didn't move freely under pressure as a lymph node would. Enlarged nodes tend to crop up in the armpit or around the elbow, not in the middle of the upper arm. The lump's redness and tenderness suggested an infection, but its firmness suggested a tumor.

The resident and I decided to take blood tests and start the girl on antibiotics in case it was a local infection. We also ordered an ultrasound examination of her arm. He would see her back in the clinic in the afternoon.

The next day the radiologist informed us that the child's lump was a lymph node, and she suspected it was enlarged due to cat scratch disease. "Cat scratch disease?" I said. "That's a surprise. I'll be right there."

Once considered rare, cat scratch disease is now known to be one of the most common causes of swollen and infected lymph nodes in children. The causative bacterium, Bartonella henselae, is commonly found in cats, especially kittens. The bacteria enter the body when a child is scratched or bitten by an infected feline. Within 3 to 10 days there may be a small red bump at the site of the scratch. Over the next few days the bacteria multiply, and the child may develop a fever, headache, or other signs of mild illness. Meanwhile, the bacteria move into the intricate network of lymph vessels, a system of channels that carry fluid, pathogens, and debris out of the tissues. The lymph node becomes large and firm as bacteria multiply and attract passing immune cells that make antibodies to the pathogen. Fortunately, cat scratch disease usually subsides without treatment.

The resident reassured the child and her mother that she would get better. He sent her to the lab for a blood test to confirm the diagnosis, which would be back in a few days. After they left, we went to see the radiologist. She pointed out the distinctive appearance of an enlarged lymph node on the ultrasound image. I realized that the extreme firmness of the node was the result of the infection's intensity and rapid progression. Still, there was one other part of the story that didn't make sense.

"I thought she hadn't had any exposure to animals," I said to the resident.

"Well, that's what she told me. Turns out she was scratched by the neighbor's kitten a couple of weeks ago."

"Let me guess," I said. "She didn't tell her mother, or us, because Mom told her not to play with the neighbor's kitten."

"That's exactly right!" he said. "How did you know?"

The radiologist and I exchanged smiles, and I turned to the young resident with a grin. "You don't have kids, do you?"

Mark Cohen is a pediatrician in Santa Clara, California.

CHAPTER

18

HIGH HEAD PRESSURE

By Mark Cohen

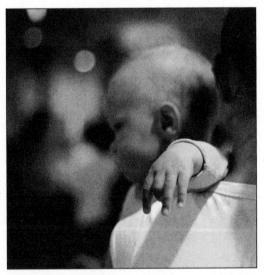

Photo 18-1

"Your next patient is ready, Dr. Cohen," the medical assistant said, placing a three-inch-thick chart on my desk. Like all the other infants I'd seen that morning, the boy was considered at high risk, and it is my job to oversee follow-up care for such patients after they leave the neonatal intensive care unit.

Now nine months old, the boy had been born very prematurely, weighing 1,400 grams—just over three pounds—at 31 weeks. According to the discharge summary, he had had mild respiratory distress syndrome, which results from immaturity of the lungs; it is one of the common complications of prematurity. But he had escaped the other major problems of premature infants, like sepsis (bloodstream infection), necrotizing enterocolitis (a serious and potentially fatal intestinal disorder), and intraventricular hemorrhage (bleeding inside the brain). When he was discharged, he was in very good shape.

Over the past eight months at home, however, he had not had an easy time. The chart notes told me that he was being treated for persistent gastroenterological reflux. Although this condition in infants is usually benign, it can sometimes cause recurrent vomiting, irritability, and failure to gain weight.

"I'm glad we also have an appointment with the gastroenterologist today," his mother said, with a worried look, "because the reflux is getting worse. He's been fussier for the past couple of weeks, and he's been vomiting much more often. He just doesn't seem like himself."

When I examined the baby, he appeared uncomfortable, and his head looked too big: the upper part of his skull appeared out of proportion to his face. That was a red flag. The rest of his examination was fairly unremarkable, although he wasn't as playful and interactive as I would have expected for an infant his age. The therapist then did a developmental assessment, which consists of playing with the baby and observing how he manipulates toys, solves simple puzzles, and so forth. Her findings confirmed that he was lagging in all areas, even after correcting for his preterm birth. The lag was particularly puzzling because the boy had done so well as a newborn.

While the therapist was doing the exam, I went back and looked at the baby's growth chart. His height and weight growth were fine, but when I plotted his head circumference, my jaw dropped. I repeated the head measurement after he was finished with the test, and I got the same number.

Up through his last visit to the pediatrician, at six months, the boy's head circumference had been following the curve between the 25th and 50th percentile. Today it was above the 95th percentile line. That was alarming. The baby's recent increase in vomiting and fussiness might have originated not in his stomach but in his head. I suspected that he had hydrocephalus, a condition in which increased cerebrospinal fluid squeezes the brain against the skull. His symptoms and his developmental delays might have been getting worse because of the increased pressure.

Hydrocephalus (a literal translation from the Greek yields the colloquial name for the condition, water on the brain) is a common complication of intraventricular bleeding in the fragile, underdeveloped brain tissue of premature infants. Even if the bleeding causes no immediate brain injury and the baby recovers, the blood that remains inside the ventricles—the fluid-filled spaces inside the brain—can sometimes block the circulation of cerebrospinal fluid, leading to a buildup of pressure. If it isn't relieved, the increasing pressure, which causes the baby's head to enlarge, can damage the brain.

From his medical records, I could see that the ultrasound scans taken while the boy was in the neonatal unit had shown no signs of bleeding in the brain. Something wasn't making sense. After telling the boy's parents about my concerns, I obtained an urgent ultrasound of his head that afternoon. The scan showed hugely enlarged ventricles, confirming the hydrocephalus diagnosis. But the ultrasound image did not tell me why the fluid was accumulating. We needed to get a CT scan in order to obtain a better picture of the brain and ventricles. The baby also needed the expertise of a neurosurgeon.

The CT also confirmed the hydrocephalus. Although the cause was not clear, the neurosurgeon felt that the boy probably had a very small intraventricular bleed while he was in the neonatal unit. The problem had not been significant enough to show up on an ultrasound, but it had been enough to block the ventricles.

To treat the hydrocephalus, a pediatric neurosurgeon inserted a thin plastic tube, called a shunt, into the ventricles. Then he connected the tube to a tiny one-way valve on the outside of the skull and threaded the tube under the baby's skin along the neck and chest. The open end of the shunt was placed in the abdomen, where the fluid could be safely reabsorbed into the bloodstream.

I was still puzzled. If the bleeding had been there all along, why had the baby's head begun to enlarge relatively recently? The neurosurgeon didn't know.

We soon found out. After the surgery for the shunt, the baby didn't seem to be recovering as quickly or fully as expected. The neurosurgeon suspected something else was going on, so he ordered another scan. The answer this time was definitive. Deep inside the baby's brain was an abnormal mass that had not been obvious on the first study. By blocking the flow of cerebrospinal fluid through the ventricles, it was causing the hydrocephalus. The next step, an MRI scan, showed that the mass was a tumor.

That explained, at last, why the boy's head had started to grow so abruptly and rapidly.

In my more than 25 years as a pediatrician, I have never ceased to be awed by the dedication and skills of pediatric neurosurgeons. They were able to remove the malignant tumor completely. But the treatment did not end there. The baby had multiple additional operations, several courses of chemotherapy, and he will require more treatment in the future, possibly including a bone marrow transplant. Once his condition stabilizes, I will be doing another developmental assessment and will continue to do so at regular intervals. So far, he's responding well to the treatment, and we're all keeping our hopes up for the future.

Medical students and pediatric residents sometimes get annoyed because I am constantly reminding them to measure the head circumference at each well-baby visit and to plot it on the growth chart. Measuring the head is one way of following the growth of a baby's brain. For this little boy, that routine procedure may have saved his life.

Mark Cohen is a pediatrician in Santa Clara, California.

CHAPTER

19

A LEG OF LEGENDARY SIZE

By Anna Reisman

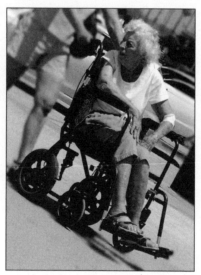

Photo 19-1

The patient was a petite 80-year-old white-haired woman in pressed Bermuda shorts. "It's nice to meet you, Mrs. Schulman," I said to her, trying my best not to gape. The medical resident,

Charles, had warned me that her leg was seriously swollen, but I still almost did a double take when I saw it.

If her left leg was a slender maple, her right was a giant redwood. It measured about three times the circumference of the left and was swollen all the way from her ankle to the very top of her thigh. It was by far the biggest swelling I'd seen in my career.

"How long has it been swollen like this?" I asked Mrs. Schulman.

"More than a month," she said. "And don't tell me to elevate it; I have it up all the time. I can't bend it, I can't garden. It's terrible!"

Charles filled me in on her medical history. She was on a blood thinner for an irregular heartbeat and a pill for high blood pressure. A few months earlier, she had tripped on a sidewalk and landed on her right knee. It still ached from time to time.

"Don't forget my cancer," Mrs. Schulman piped in. "I had lung cancer five years ago, and I beat it!"

Alarmed, I willed my eyebrows not to rise. It was painfully obvious that she might be wrong. Since cancer increases the risk of blood clots, a single swollen leg in a patient with a history of cancer was a blood clot until proved otherwise. I could see from Charles's widened eyes that he hadn't known about her cancer history until that moment.

It was possible we were wrong, of course. Swelling in one leg can also result from muscle injury, veins that no longer function properly, cysts behind the knee, infections, or a variety of knee abnormalities. But since a history of cancer and trauma are both risk factors for blood clots, we decided to start there.

Haltingly, Charles explained to our patient that she would need an ultrasound, which can often pick up a clot, and that it was important to get it immediately.

"If this is a DVT—deep vein thrombosis—a blood clot in one of your leg veins," he told her, "it could become dislodged and land in one of your lung vessels and cause a pulmonary embolus, a blockage of arteries in the lung. It could be life threatening." It's estimated that between 300,000 and 600,000 people in the United States have DVTs and pulmonary emboli each year, and 60,000 to 100,000 die from these conditions.

But Mrs. Schulman was a step ahead. She had already seen a doctor two weeks earlier who was clearly thinking along the same lines we were: he had sent her for an ultrasound, which turned out to be normal. He had also ordered a CT scan of her abdomen to evaluate her pelvic veins, where the ultrasound couldn't reach. But that was normal too. With no sign of a blood clot in either test, there was less reason to worry about a recurrence of cancer, but we still had to figure out the problem with her leg.

I suggested that we repeat the ultrasound, because sometimes blood clots don't show up immediately. An hour later, we had the result: again, no clot.

This wasn't turning out to be a cut-and-dried case after all. A hugely swollen leg in an elderly woman with a history of cancer had seemed so likely to be a blood clot, but two ultrasounds and a CT scan later, we had found nothing.

Mrs. Schulman was convinced that her knee was the problem. After her fall, she told us, her knee had been swollen for a week or so. It improved, although it still ached if she walked a lot. The massive leg swelling started more than a month later. But when I called the doctor who had seen her, he thought it unlikely that a fall could have caused this extreme degree of swelling.

Mrs. Schulman asked if an antibiotic might help. I explained to her that there was no sign of infection. Her white blood cell count, which would increase in an infection, was completely normal, and the leg did not have the increased warmth or redness that might suggest an infection of the skin or soft tissues. Instead, I suggested trying a diuretic, a medicine that helps reduce the amount of water in the body, for a week. In some cases swollen legs are simply due to water retention from poorly functioning veins. I didn't think there was much chance that was the case here, since both legs would most likely be swollen. Still, a diuretic probably wouldn't hurt.

We sent her home, but not without some trepidation. We warned her about symptoms of a blood clot in the leg, such as redness, warmth, or tenderness, or—in a worst-case scenario— the chest pain, rapid heartbeat, or shortness of breath that would result from a pulmonary embolus. Later that afternoon, still worried, I spoke with a radiologist who recommended an MRI of her leg and pelvis. Perhaps there was something obstructing the veins that hadn't been visible on either the ultrasound or the CT scan. Anything that blocks or diminishes blood flow—a blood clot within the vein, a mass pressing on the outside of the vein, damage to the vein itself—can build up pressure that is transmitted to the capillaries, causing swelling.

I called Mrs. Schulman and apologized, explaining that I was recommending yet another test, an MRI. I told her that there was a good chance that this one would give us an answer. She was eager to do whatever it took. A week later, we had the results: no blockages visible in the blood vessels, and no compression of the veins.

Desperate to find the problem, caught up in a cascade of testing, and frustrated that after more than a month her leg remained worryingly swollen, I persuaded myself to keep looking for a hidden blood clot. So I ordered a venogram, in which a contrast dye is injected into a vein and a series of X-rays depicts the flow of the dye—or, if there's an obstruction, a lack of flow. Although it is the gold standard for diagnosing deep vein thrombosis, a venogram comes with the risk of serious allergic reaction to the dye. I also consulted an oncologist, who sent Mrs. Schulman for another CT scan as well as a positron emission tomography (PET) scan, which uses small amounts of radioactive substances to generate three-dimensional images of metabolic processes within tissue and organs. Three tests and one consultant later, we had found no blood clot and no cancer, and were no closer to an answer for her swollen leg.

Mrs. Schulman made the best of life with a huge, stiff leg. She lifted it carefully when climbing stairs and she didn't plant a garden that spring. In the summer, she visited her family out of town for a few weeks. Still very worried about a blood clot, I left a series of messages for her, asking her to call when she returned. When I didn't hear back, I wondered if a clot had barreled through her veins to her lungs, and if she had ended up hospitalized or dead. Or maybe she had gone to another doctor who had solved the mystery, and she had decided never to see me (or Charles) again.

About a month later, she finally picked up the phone. "It's better," she said, cheerful as ever.

My heart lifted. "You mean, the swelling is down a little?"

"No, it's back to normal. Same size as the other one."

My mouth dropped open. Mrs. Schulman told me she'd taken an antibiotic prescribed by her other doctor for the knee pain, and within a week, the swelling had melted away.

I called her doctor, eager to hear the story. He'd thrown up his hands, he told me. So many tests, no answers, and a patient who had wanted an antibiotic from day one. It made no sense, he said, but why the heck not.

Though it was possible she had an infection whose signs we missed and that the antibiotic cleared up, my take was that it was a coincidence. Some antibiotics have anti-inflammatory effects on arthritis when used over time, but I didn't think arthritis was the underlying cause of her leg swelling either.

Even though Mrs. Schulman recovered in the aftermath of antibiotic treatment, I wasn't convinced it made a difference. Whatever made the swelling subside was as mysterious as whatever had caused it.

In up to a quarter of the cases of single-leg swelling with negative venograms, no precise cause is ever identified. Plenty of questions cannot be answered by diagnostic tests, and often, symptoms fade before we can pinpoint their exact cause. Time may not heal all wounds, but as far as I am concerned, it worked for this one.

Anna Reisman is an internist in West Haven, Connecticut.

CHAPTER

20

THE SNEAKY PAIN THAT FOOLED 6 EXPERTS

By Anna Reisman

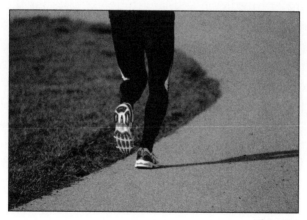

Photo 20-1

Forty-two-year-old Russell McCoy was energized and sweaty as he finished a three-mile run around his neighborhood. He headed straight for his refrigerator and cracked open a diet soda, downing it in a couple of swigs. Holding the empty can, he backed toward the garbage pail, pivoted, shot, and scored. Then pain, sudden and excruciating, lanced through his left hip. He bent over, aware that he had twisted something the wrong way. Breathing deeply, he felt a little better. A few hours later, though, he tried to run a few strides and almost yelped from the pain. For the next two weeks, he took it easy. But the hip didn't get better.

I first saw Mr. McCoy in June, two months after the soda can episode. He had already been to another doctor, who was convinced this was "referred pain"—in other words, pain in one body area that is actually the result of a problem in another. According to that doctor, Mr. McCoy had strained his lower back muscles and was experiencing it as hip pain. A week of anti-inflammatory medicine and stretching exercises for the lower back had not helped, however. An X-ray of the hip a month later showed no sign of arthritis or fracture, and an MRI of the lower back hadn't revealed much either, just a small disk bulge that seemed unrelated to the pain.

My patient told me that, over the two months since the injury, he had gained 10 pounds. He wasn't exercising because it hurt too much. He wasn't sleeping well, either; the hip ached when he lay on his left side. He sucked his breath in sharply when I pushed on the greater trochanter, the bony outer part of his upper left thigh.

His main symptom—the sore spot on his hip that hurt when pressed—was typical for trochanteric bursitis, inflammation of the greater trochanter's bursa. A bursa is a fluid-filled sac that allows adjacent tissues to glide over each other. When injury or overuse irritates the bursa, any pressure or movement around it will cause pain. I recommended treating the inflammation with a cortisone injection.

My patient cringed at the thought of a needle poking into the painful area. Instead, he decided to seek yet another opinion, this time from an orthopedic surgeon. Like the first doctor, the surgeon believed the symptoms originated in the lower back. He had Mr. McCoy see a physical therapist, who thought the back had nothing to do with it and that he had strained a muscle in his hip. The next stop was a chiropractor, who worked on both hip and back with no improvement.

Finally, four months after our first visit, Mr. McCoy was back in my waiting room. His belly now bulged over his belt, and he grimaced each time his left foot hit the floor. "I'm ready for the injection," he said. "Let's go for it."

I had him lie on his right side, located the tenderest area on the top of his left thigh, and injected a mixture of anesthetic and cortisone. Injections like these are among the few procedures that can give almost instant relief. The anesthetic numbs the sore area immediately, and the steroid kicks in within two days. If the anesthetic helped, it would support my diagnosis, and we could be pretty sure that the steroid would work. If the anesthetic didn't help, then it probably wasn't trochanteric bursitis after all.

I held my breath as he took a few steps. He winced. The injection had not worked.

It had been six months since Mr. McCoy first hurt his hip, and now we were right back where we started. I had run out of ideas. The physical exam, the X-ray results, and the injection had ruled out the common causes of hip pain—arthritis, bursitis, fracture, referred pain from the lower back—but he still couldn't run. In many situations, the search for a cause of pain ends without an answer, and we change our focus to pain control. But I was not ready to give up.

Apologizing for adding yet another doctor into the mix, I suggested a rheumatologist—a joint specialist—who then sent Mr. McCoy for a procedure in which an anesthetic, followed by cortisone, was injected directly into the ball-and-socket part of the hip joint. This, too, failed to relieve the pain.

We had not yet addressed the slight disk bulge that appeared on the MRI of Mr. McCoy's lower back. I didn't think it was the culprit, but we had no other leads. Disk bulges are notoriously tricky to interpret because they are common in people both with and without pain; in fact, they appear on MRIs of people without back pain roughly 50 percent of the time. So it isn't easy to decide whether a bulge justifies the discomfort, expense, and radiation exposure of additional tests, or even surgery.

Mr. McCoy's neurosurgery appointment wouldn't happen for another two months. While he waited, I suggested he return to the physical therapist for a cane and some hip exercises.

When I saw him a month later, in January, I had to blink a couple of times. He wasn't limping. He wasn't using a cane. He was smiling.

What he told me was so utterly unexpected, so simple, that I was at a loss for words. "I have a short leg," he explained. "The physical therapist measured my legs, and my right one is about half an inch shorter. He gave me a heel lift and it's working like a charm."

I had not learned about leg length discrepancy (LLD) in my training, and it seemed that none of the other clinicians Mr. McCoy saw had considered it either. But leg length discrepancies are common. According to some studies, up to 70 percent of people have a slight difference in the length of their legs; one person in a thousand has a difference of nearly an inch. In most cases, the difference goes undetected.

There are two kinds of LLD. Structural discrepancies, which can be congenital or the result of a fracture or hip replacement surgery, involve an actual difference in the length of the bones. Functional discrepancies, on the other hand, are caused by muscle weakness or stiffness in the pelvis, ankle, or foot—the legs are the same size but function as if one is longer. Mr. McCoy probably had a lifelong mild leg length discrepancy that never bothered him until he hurt his hip. The pain changed the way he walked, and all of a sudden the discrepancy mattered.

My patient's LLD was small enough that it had never caused an obvious limp, at least until now. But there was another clue that nobody had noticed. "I looked at the soles of his shoes, and one was more worn," the physical therapist told me. "If the right leg is shorter, you tend to walk on the outer part of that foot, to extend the leg. On the other side, to make the longer leg feel shorter, you flatten out that foot. You can learn a lot from the soles."

One common method used to check for a structural leg length discrepancy involves running a tape measure from a point on the pelvis to the ankle bone several times and then averaging the numbers. To check for a functional discrepancy, a physical therapist will measure from the belly button to each ankle bone. Some doctors recommend taking a special X-ray to verify the measurement; others believe that the degree of accuracy achieved with an X-ray is not worth the radiation exposure and is not necessary with small discrepancies.

Physical therapists often give a patient with hip pain and a small LLD a heel lift or even an insert from a sneaker to try for a week or so. What makes the treatment tricky is that a heel lift doesn't always work. As with those incidental disk bulges on MRIs, a leg length discrepancy may have nothing to do with the pain; since a slight difference in leg lengths is so common, it would be easy to make the mistake of treating the pain with a heel lift when there is another reason for it, like arthritis or bursitis. And some people have had an LLD for so long that they've compensated by holding their pelvis at a certain angle. In those situations, a heel lift that is used for more than a week may end up causing pain rather than relieving it.

For some people, the search for relief from hip pain never ends. Luckily, that wasn't the case with my patient. The heel lift did more than match the length of his legs. It lifted his spirits.

Anna Reisman is an internist in West Haven, Connecticut.

CHAPTER

21

ONE CURE FOR VERTIGO: PLAYING PINBALL INSIDE YOUR HEAD

By Anna Reisman

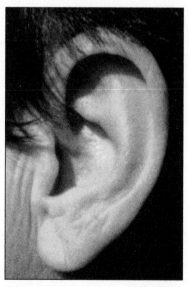

Photo 21-1

Thomas Riccio, a lanky 84-year-old, was dozing off in the waiting room. A former crane operator at a steel mill and a World War II veteran, he had been in for a physical six months earlier and everything was fine. His only chronic medical problem was high blood pressure.

When I called his name, he stood up and swayed, almost losing his balance. His wife and I lunged, each grabbing one of his arms.

"I'm okay, I'm okay," he insisted. "Just when I get up sometimes, I almost lose my balance, but I haven't fallen."

His wife told me it was the fourth time in three months that he'd come to the VA (Veterans Affairs) clinic with dizziness. At our regular visits he always said that everything was good. He wasn't one to complain.

Slowly we made our way down the hall, Mr. Riccio sliding one hand along the wall.

Dizziness is the third most common symptom in primary care, and it's one that doctors love to hate. That is because each of the three main categories of dizziness—vertigo, disequilibrium, and light-headedness—has its own lengthy list of diagnoses.

Vertigo is an illusory sensation of motion or spinning, often accompanied by nausea. It can be caused by inner-ear problems, migraines, or, if accompanied by other symptoms, a stroke. Disequilibrium—which is particularly common in elderly patients with arthritis or problems with vision, hearing, or balance—is a feeling of unsteadiness while walking unaided across an open space. Light-headedness is the sensation of nearly fainting, such as one might experience when standing up suddenly after a day of gardening in the hot sun. It most often results from problems in blood flow to the brain caused by anemia, low blood sugar, hyperventilation, dehydration, or cardiac problems.

Which of these three was Mr. Riccio experiencing? I wasn't the first doctor to consider the question. Mr. Riccio told me he had gone to the emergency room three months earlier, complaining of dizziness and headaches he'd had off and on for several days. Given the patient's history of high blood pressure, the emergency room doctor suspected a stroke, so he asked for a CT scan of Mr. Riccio's brain to see if there were any blocked or burst blood vessels. He also requested blood tests for signs of anemia or low blood sugar. The CT scan and the blood work both came back normal. Mr. Riccio was discharged with instructions to take Tylenol, in case he was experiencing a migraine. During the next three weeks, both the headache and the dizziness eased, but then the dizziness returned.

Over the next few months, he saw three more doctors. One ascribed the headache and dizziness to sinusitis. Another thought it could be inflammation of the inner ear. Another believed elevated blood pressure was the cause. Mr. Riccio tried various treatments to no avail.

Now it was my chance to solve the puzzle.

"It comes and goes," Mr. Riccio told me. "Last night in bed, I thought I was going to pass out. The room suddenly whizzed around. Just for about 10 seconds, but it felt a lot longer."

Did it happen more if he turned his head to one side or the other?

He thought for a moment. "To the right," he said. "When I turn my head to the right fast, I get dizzy."

"When you stood up in the waiting room, you looked pretty dizzy," I said. "When you stand up fast, do you usually get kind of light-headed, like you're going to faint?"

He shook his head.

What happened when he walked across a large open space? Did he feel unsteady? He said that he didn't.

I asked Mr. Riccio to follow my forefinger with his eyes. A jerking in his eye movements when he tracked my finger could indicate a problem with the balancing system of the inner ear. The other doctors hadn't noted any rhythmic jerkiness, called nystagmus, but I wanted to double-check. I repeated the test a couple of times. Mr. Riccio's eye movements were smooth.

Sometimes the information we get from a patient's history doesn't match up with the physical, and we have to go with our gut feeling. My gut was telling me that this was vertigo, even without nystagmus. Could it be benign paroxysmal positional vertigo (BPPV)? This is the most common type of positional vertigo, and it occurs most frequently in the elderly. In almost half of all cases, there is no known cause.

There is one leading hypothesis about how it happens. Inside the inner ear are three fluid-filled, semicircular canals that serve as balance sensors. In patients with BPPV, tiny chunks of calcium carbonate crystals, called otoconia, float into the canals. The crystals are normally attached to a membrane in the inner ear, but they can be dislodged, perhaps by head injury or infection or through the normal degeneration of aging.

"You know those little handheld pinball games?" I asked. Mr. Riccio nodded. "The crystals are like the tiny metal balls in one of those games. Once they're in the wrong spot, it's hard to get them back. They roll around every time you move your head and unintentionally set off motion sensors. So your brain gets the wrong information about balance. It thinks you're moving in one direction when you're really not. So it overcorrects, and you end up with the spinning sensation."

He leaned forward and pursed his lips.

"Is there another pill to try?" He sounded tired, a little frustrated.

"Something even better."

In 1983, John Epley, an otolaryngologist in Portland, Oregon, found that a precise series of guided head movements could rid patients of vertigo by directing the disruptive crystals out of the semicircular canals. Initially the local medical community dismissed his finding. To many physicians, any technique based on a maneuver or manipulation smacks of hocus-pocus. But the treatment was backed up by scientific studies, and by 1992 doctors had come to accept it.

The Epley maneuver is now the standard treatment for BPPV. Because it involves manipulating the head and neck into certain positions, in rare instances it is not recommended for patients with unstable heart disease, severe blockage of the carotid arteries, or neck disease. Otherwise the maneuver is safe and quite effective, relieving vertigo in 80 percent of patients with BPPV.

It was worth a try.

I asked Mr. Riccio to sit on the exam table again. I explained that we needed to position him so he was lying on his back with his head hanging to one side and gently tilted backward. I warned him that the changes in position would momentarily trigger the dizziness, if my suspicion about the cause of his vertigo was correct.

Standing at his side, I said, "Hold my right forearm," as I braced my left hand on his back. "Now turn your head to the right and keep it turned as you lie down." I guided him down until he was flat on his back, his head tilted back over the edge, his right ear pointing at the floor.

"Whoa, there it goes," he said, opening his eyes wide. "That's the feeling. That's the one." As I moved his head into the different positions, I pictured a little pinball game and imagined I was directing the tiny balls—the crystals—back into their designated holes.

After 30 seconds I turned his head gently so his left ear was pointing down. Then I instructed him to keep his head still and to roll over onto his left shoulder, keeping his head angled down to the exam table. Another 30 seconds.

"Now please sit up without changing the position of your head and tell me if you still feel dizzy." I helped him up.

"Oh yeah, very dizzy." He braced himself, clutching the edge of the exam table.

We repeated the whole sequence two more times, and by the last time Mr. Riccio sat up, the dizziness was gone. It might come back, I told him, but it would probably be less intense. I printed a diagram showing how he could do a modified version of the Epley maneuver at home, using a pillow under the shoulders to position his head at the correct angle. If he did this a few times a day until the dizziness was gone for 24 hours, it would probably stay away for a while, and in some cases for good.

Two months later he was back for his regular checkup. We walked briskly from the waiting room to my office. He was beaming.

"Doctor, can I give you a hug?" he asked. "You cured me!"

Just call me a pinball wizard.

Anna Reisman is an internist in West Haven, Connecticut.

CHAPTER

22

CRUISING INTO TROUBLE

By Anna Reisman

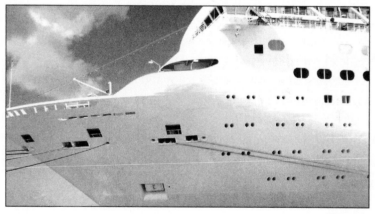

Photo 22-1

"Your admission is Evelyn Warwick, little old lady in distress." The emergency room resident motioned toward a curtained area at the far end of the ward. "Completely delirious."

"Got it," I said. At the time I was a medical resident at a New York City public hospital, supervising an intern and a medical student. I knew that delirium, an acute confusional state, could result from just about any type of acute illness, or it could be a side effect of medication. And yet, I explained to my team, you could often guess the cause simply from the type of patient.

We all agreed about Mrs. Warwick's probable diagnosis. An elderly woman with delirium at a public city hospital was likely to be a nursing home patient with pneumonia or a urinary tract infection. She might be dehydrated, or maybe she'd had a stroke or a heart attack.

When I pulled back the curtain, I did a double take. Evelyn Warwick was a handsome woman with a neat gray bob like an elementary school principal, not a typical city hospital patient. Her pink pajamas glowed against the starched white sheets. Mr. Warwick, a silver-haired man in a tweed jacket, stroked her forehead with a damp cloth.

I introduced myself and the team and asked how she was feeling. She opened her watery blue eyes and stared far into the distance. "I don't know where I am!" she murmured in a clipped British accent. "I woke up and my head exploded." She looked around the room in a panic and started to weep. "Where am I? What's all this?"

Her husband patted her hand. "We were on the QE2, darling. Four days at sea since we left Southampton. We docked in New York yesterday, remember? You woke up in the hotel. . . . You were so upset." Mrs. Warwick closed her eyes and sighed.

"At three in the morning, she bolted up and woke me in a fright," her husband continued. "She didn't know where she was."

She had no medical history of note and took only a daily vitamin. She didn't drink, Mr. Warwick told us, no more than a glass of white wine with dinner. Except for a mild fever and a slightly rapid heart rate, her physical exam was normal. Her blood and urine tests, so far, were unremarkable: She wasn't anemic, her electrolytes were fine, and she wasn't dehydrated. An electrocardiogram showed no evidence of a heart attack. She'd had a normal chest X-ray, and a CT scan of her brain hadn't shown any sign of a stroke or tumor. The initial results of her spinal tap were normal too.

I laid my hand on hers, which was warm, sweaty, and jittery, and asked her if she had felt any different in the last few days. Her eyes popped open and darted back and forth. "I don't know, I don't know where I am!" she said, her face creased with worry.

"You're at a hospital," I reminded her. "We're going to help you feel better, I promise."

Mr. Warwick scratched his head. "She did say she felt a little under the weather. Nothing out of the ordinary." He watched his wife turn her head from side to side and ask again where she was. "Last night we had a late dinner at the hotel," he told me. "She had some broth, a little salad, half a glass of wine. She didn't have much appetite, a bit of a headache. Didn't think much of it, after such a long journey."

So far, her symptoms and test results hadn't given up any clues. I left the room, hoisted a few textbooks over to the doctor's station, and started to read. We'd ruled out the most common causes of delirium, but I wanted to make sure I wasn't missing anything.

Then I came upon a syndrome I'd never heard of before: transient global amnesia. TGA, I read, usually occurs in older people and often produces a brief period of anterograde amnesia, the inability to form new memories. Patients often ask about the date and place again and again, and they sometimes experience headache and nausea. Even though TGA is rare—each year, it affects up to 32 per 100,000 people over age 50—and is typically brought on by strenuous activity, I realized it might explain Mrs. Warwick's symptoms. Maybe the long voyage had been too much for a 65-year-old woman. If this really was TGA, she should be better within 24 hours.

I paged my intern and student and we went to get a snack from the vending machines. I told them about TGA, and they agreed that the diagnosis made sense. But when we got back to the ER, a nurse waved us over urgently. "I just paged you," she said. "Mrs. Warwick's temperature spiked to 103 and she's hallucinating, very agitated. I don't know where the husband is."

We rushed back to the bedside. So much for transient global amnesia. Mrs. Warwick was thrashing around on the bed as though possessed. Sweat poured down her face, and her blood pressure had skyrocketed. "She just pulled out her IV," the nurse explained. "She needs restraints, okay?"

"Fine." My heart thudded in my ears. I couldn't think. Mrs. Warwick cursed and hollered gibberish as the nurse wrapped restraints around her wrists and tied them to the bedrails.

Someone was tapping my shoulder. "Shouldn't we give her some benzos?" Jeff, the medical student, was asking. I took a deep breath and refocused. I explained that in most cases of delirium, benzodiazepines—antianxiety medicines that include diazepam (Valium)—can actually worsen symptoms. Instead, I asked the nurse to give her haloperidol (Haldol), an antipsychotic that can safely calm a delirious patient.

The Haldol wouldn't take effect for at least 30 minutes. I feared that Mrs. Warwick would go into cardiac arrest or have an arrhythmia or a stroke or be overwhelmed by infection, and I didn't know what else to do. We were going nowhere with our diagnoses while my patient was plummeting downhill.

Leah, the intern, interrupted my frantic thoughts. "I keep think-ing this looks like DT," she said. "Though I know it can't be . . ."

DT is an abbreviation for delirium tremens, a life-threatening state that affects 5 percent of people withdrawing from alcohol. People with DT are disoriented, sweaty, and febrile, and they sometimes hallucinate. Dangerous cardiac arrhythmias and respiratory failure can lead to death. A century ago, 37 percent of people with DT died; nowadays, due to better treatment, it is about 5 percent.

"You can't have DT with one glass of wine a day," I said, my mind furiously trying to piece things together.

Mr. Warwick walked back in at that moment. He was shocked to find his wife tied to the bed, wailing. He demanded to know what was going on. I gulped and hoped what I was about to say wouldn't offend him. "I know you said your wife didn't drink much, but she looks like she might be withdrawing from alcohol. Is it possible that she drinks more than you told us?"

He stared at me, his face blank, and I started to apologize. But then he lifted a hand. "Truth is, she drinks a lot." Tears formed in his eyes. "Much more in the last three years, since she retired. She drinks when I'm at work. She thinks it's a secret. I thought she'd stop on the cruise, since we'd be together all the time. I didn't know stopping could make her so ill."

Now things were starting to make sense. "So she was drinking a lot, and then on the cruise she was having only one drink a day, for the last four days." I was thinking out loud. "She felt poorly because she was starting to go into alcohol withdrawal. And now she's in delirium tremens."

I turned to my team and the nurse. "We need to get benzos on board—now."

The nurse hurried off, and the medical student looked confused. "But you said they were dangerous in delirium."

I explained that in alcohol withdrawal syndromes, benzodiazepines can be lifesaving. Neurons in the brain strive to maintain a balance (homeostasis) between sedation and excitement. There are two main types of neurotransmitters involved. GABA is inhibitory and causes sedation; glutamate, its opposite, is excitatory. Specific receptors on the neurons detect GABA (the GABA receptor) and glutamate (the NMDA receptor). Alcohol is sensed through the GABA receptor. Like GABA, it enhances sedation. In a chronic drinker, the presence of all that sedating alcohol in the body means that the neurons don't need so many GABA receptors. They cut down on those and create more excitatory NMDA receptors.

When a chronic drinker abruptly stops drinking, the balance is thrown off. With fewer inhibiting GABA receptors and more excitatory NMDA/glutamate receptors, the neurons become overstimulated. In mild alcohol withdrawal, a person will become jittery, anxious, and irritable; in DT, the person's system will go haywire. Benzodiazepines, like alcohol, work at the GABA receptor and induce a sedated and safer state. The benzodiazepines can then be tapered off gradually while the brain resets its balance.

When Mrs. Warwick left the hospital five days later, she was back to normal, minus any plans to drink alcohol ever again. "Scared straight," the medical student remarked after the Warwicks headed back to England. That would be great, I told him, but I knew she would probably drink again if she didn't seek help.

The key to preventing DT in any hospitalized patient with a drinking problem is giving benzodiazepines as soon as possible.

But doing so depends on our ability to recognize a patient at risk. Too often we overlook the diagnosis in people who don't look like alcoholics—especially older women, up to 8 percent of whom have an alcohol problem.

Sometimes a missed drink, whether missed by the drinker or by the doctor, can be a matter of life and death.

Anna Reisman is an internist in West Haven, Connecticut.

CHAPTER

23

THE WOMAN WHO NEEDED TO BE UPSIDE-DOWN

By Louis F. Janeira

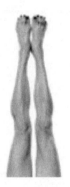

Photo 23-1

The emergency room was busy that afternoon. I had just started my shift and was making my way through a scrum of frantic doctors, nurses, and orderlies when I heard yelling coming from the ambulance bay entrance.

"Put her down now!" I recognized the stern voice of Herb, one of our security guards.

"Get a stretcher, stat," said Ellie, the head nurse.

"You're hurting her," a woman yelled.

I ran to the ambulance bay, rounded a corner, and saw a huge man, 7-foot-something, holding a petite woman, maybe five feet tall, by her feet, her head dangling down. "I have to hold her this way," the man insisted.

"I'm fine," said the woman through her dangling long black hair. "I feel okay now."

Herb grabbed at the man's muscular arms, attempting to free the woman.

"This is my wife," the giant shouted. "Let go of me." He glared at Herb, who kept pulling at his biceps and wrists. A large group of ER personnel was now watching them from a distance.

"Let's everybody take a deep breath here," I said. "What's your name, sir?"

Herb released his grip on the man and took a step back.

"Jason," he said, more calmly now.

"Okay, Jason," I said. "Why are you carrying your wife by her feet?"

"Hi, Dr. Janeira," said the upside-down woman. "Remember me?"

"No," I said. "Have we met?"

"Yes, I was here yesterday," she said. "Remember? With the slow heartbeat?"

And then it came to me. Her name was Mary, a woman in her mid-60s. She had arrived at the ER the day before with complete heart block, caused when the electrical system connecting the atria to the ventricles fails because of scarring, infection, or heart attack. As a result, the heart slows dramatically.

Mary's heart rate had been under 40 beats per minute instead of the 60 to 80 that would be considered normal in her age group.

She was having recurrent fainting spells and seizures. This giant hadn't been with her then, and I had called a colleague for urgent implantation of a pacemaker, which generates rhythmic electrical pulses that prevent slowing of the heartbeat. Within minutes she had been taken from my ER to a laboratory where she was fitted for the device.

I approached the couple slowly. "I didn't expect to see you so soon," I said leaning over, trying to see her face. "Didn't you have your pacemaker implanted yesterday?"

"Yes," she said. "I had the surgery yesterday. Everything went well, and I went home this morning."

"Everything was good until about half an hour ago," Jason said. "She coughed and then collapsed."

"But I don't understand why you're keeping her upside down," I said.

"I picked her up and put her on our bed," Jason explained. "She regained consciousness for a few seconds. She tried to get up but went out again and fell behind the bed. I picked her up by her ankles and she came to."

"I still don't get it," I said.

"If Jason puts me in bed or upright, I faint again," Mary told me. "We've tried it four times now, and every time he changes my position, I go to la-la land."

"So you're conscious upside down but not right side up?" I asked.

Mary's upside-down head nodded vigorously.

AN URGENT DIAGNOSIS

My mind raced through the possibilities. Mary could have something obstructing the blood flow from her heart to her brain that was overcome when her head was down. Or her blood pressure could be so low that blood reached the brain only when she was upside down. Blood pressure that low could have been triggered by an allergic reaction, anaphylactic shock, or severe dehydration.

Another possibility was that Mary was suffering from cardiac tamponade, a compression of the heart caused by a buildup of blood in the sac covering the organ. If her heart had been perforated during the pacemaker implantation and blood had seeped out into the sac around it, it might be that her ventricles were now being squeezed by this accumulating blood, lowering her cardiac output. That condition could improve when she was upside down by increasing blood flow to the brain.

The first thing to do was to check Mary's vital signs. "Bring her into a room," I said.

"Let's get her on a monitor."

I pointed the way, and Jason carried her into the cardiac room, an entourage of curious ER personnel trailing behind us.

Even once in the cardiac room, Jason was unconvinced that he should let go of her ankles and put her on the bed. "When I put her down, she'll go out on us," he said.

I paused for a moment. "We'll do an assessment of the vital signs first while Mary is upside down. Then we'll put her in bed and see if and how things change, OK?"

Jason nodded. Mary's long black hair waved back and forth, which I took for agreement from her, too. Ellie then placed heart monitor electrodes on her chest.

"Normal-paced rhythm," I said, watching the monitor. "The pacemaker is working perfectly fine right now."

"And I feel perfectly fine," said Mary. "Well, except that I'm upside down and have been for about 30 minutes now."

Ellie wrapped a blood pressure cuff around her arm. "It's 120 over 66," said Ellie. "Pretty good."

"OK, slowly get her on her back," I said. Jason walked closer to the bed and Ellie and I eased Mary down onto it. The only sound came from the heart monitor: beep, beep, beep, steady at 60 times a minute. We all held our breath.

Then the cardiac monitor showed a sudden change. The alarm began screaming.

"Here I go," said Mary. "It's happeni . . ." Her words dissolved into nothingness.

"No heart rhythm," Ellie called out. "Pacemaker failure."

"Get me epinephrine," I yelled. Also known as adrenaline, epinephrine is a hormone that can constrict blood vessels and get a stalled heart beating again.

"But we don't have an IV in yet," said Ellie.

"Out of my way," said Jason, pushing us aside to get to Mary's feet. "I told you this would happen." The big man grabbed Mary's ankles and pulled them up in the air. Moments after Mary was upside down again, the heart monitor resumed steadily beeping.

"I'm back," said Mary.

Something must have gone wrong with her operation yesterday, I thought. Then suddenly it hit me. "The pacemaker lead, the wire going from the pacemaker generator to your right ventricle, must have disconnected. Your coughing spell could have done it," I said. "Somehow, the lead reconnects when you are upside down and continues to stimulate the heart."

Pacemakers are made up of two main components, a generator and a lead that carries electrical impulses to the heart. Often the lead tip is screwed directly into the heart muscle, but in rare cases it can dislodge and cease to stimulate the heart. Data from

St. Jude Medical, one of the largest pacemaker manufacturers, show that out of about 220,000 implants of the company's most popular lead attached directly to the heart, only 97 dislodged within 30 days of implantation. Apparently, Mary was one of the rare cases.

GETTING THE PATIENT UPRIGHT

"How are we going to fix this, Doc?" Jason wanted to know.

"You'll need to go back to surgery to reattach the lead," I said to Mary. "Let's page your electrophysiologist stat." I looked at Jason and sighed. "Meanwhile, keep her upside down."

We inserted an IV in Mary's arm and hooked her up to an external pacing device. But pacing her heart through her chest wall gave her severe discomfort and was not a good option, even in the short term. Moreover, it turned out that Mary's slow beat did not respond at all to medications, including intravenous epinephrine. So she was quickly transported to the electrophysiology laboratory, dangling by her ankles, carried by the only man around with enough strength to do it. And my ER shift continued.

The next day I was back on duty. As I came out of a room after examining a small child with a fever, I heard a familiar voice behind me.

"Dr. Janeira, it's me, Mary. I'm all fixed up."

I turned and smiled at Mary and nodded at Jason, who towered massively behind her.

"You were right. The pacemaker's ventricular lead had to be re-screwed in my heart," she said. "I'll be having the pacemaker checked in a few days and then every three months."

"How do you feel now?" I asked.

"Back to normal," she said. "Thanks for your help!"

And with that, she left my ER walking upright and hand-in-hand with her giant.

Louis F. Janeira is a cardiac electrophysiologist in Terre Haute, Indiana.

CHAPTER

24

THE PATIENT'S SYMPTOMS RESEMBLED A BACKACHE, BUT THEIR CAUSE MIGHT PROVE FAR MORE DEADLY

By Tony Dajer

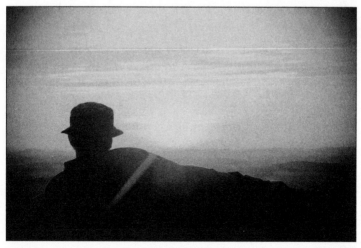

Photo 24-1

He caught my eye the minute he strolled into the emergency room, just before midnight. He had wrapped both hands around his lower back and kept straightening up, as if to work out a kink. The resident examined him first.

"Seventy-one-year-old man with back pain," he reported. "Began six hours ago, and it's getting worse. Funny thing is, he didn't lift anything heavy, or fall. Should I give him something for the pain?"

"Can you find where it hurts?" I asked.

"I checked along his back. Nothing."

"Pulses?" I continued.

He frowned. "I forgot to check."

"Maybe," I said, "it isn't his back."

I went over to say hi. The patient had the weathered mien of a smoker.

"Hello, Doctor," he said in a gravelly voice. "I need something for this pain."

I pressed up and down his back: no sore muscles or tender vertebrae. His belly hurt a little in the left lower quadrant. Above his navel, I felt carefully for a pulsing, painful fullness but found none. The pulses in his groin seemed a little uneven—the right stronger than the left—but I couldn't be sure. Most intriguing was the appearance of his legs. A lacy pattern of blue seemed to play over them, a mottling that suggested his blood wasn't circulating well.

"I'm not sure what's causing your pain," I confessed. "Until I am, I can't give you anything for the pain. It would only mask things."

"It hurts. Hurts like a bear, Doctor."

"Soon as I can. I promise."

The resident and I stepped away.

"What are you thinking?" he asked.

"Triple-A: abdominal aortic aneurysm."

"But shouldn't we be able to feel it?"

"Not always. He needs a diagnosis," I said. "Preferably in the next five minutes."

It's easy to forget that the aorta arches off the heart, diving down through the diaphragm and running along the left side of the spinal column. At the level of the navel, it forks into two big arteries, the iliacs, to feed the lower body. Buried beneath the abdominal wall and the intestines, shielded from the rear by ribs and back muscles, the abdominal aorta lies at our very pith. Thick and resilient, it swells with every squeeze of the heart's left ventricle, then smoothly recoils to keep the pressure wave moving along. This elasticity is its Achilles' heel. Age, combined more often than not with the insults of cigarette smoking and atherosclerosis, can weaken the aortic wall in the upper abdomen until it balloons like a worn inner tube.

When an aneurysm gets too big or too weak, it bursts. If the tear is recognized and repaired immediately, about half of these patients survive. But aneurysms can also leak, ooze, or expand in so many ways that a good third of them end up misdiagnosed. Clinicians often expect to find a tender mass in the upper abdomen, but that clue isn't always present. Worse, the belly may not be particularly sensitive to an examining hand. In fact, aneurysms are usually asymptomatic until they start leaking, especially in overweight patients. As the blood oozes slowly into the tough tissues around the spinal cord, the symptoms can mimic anything from a kidney stone to diverticulitis to a slipped disk.

To exclude the possibility of an aneurysm, you need an ultrasound or a CAT scan. My hospital has no ultrasound at night, and the CAT scan was down. Moreover, our operating room could not handle major vascular surgery.

My hazy impression would have to do: He had to be transferred fast.

I called uptown for the vascular surgery resident. It took 10 minutes to get an operator, then another 10 for a sleepy voice to answer. "Vascular."

"Hi, this is Dr. Dajer," I said. "I've got a 71-year-old man, smoker, with increasingly severe back pain for six hours. His abdomen shows left lower quadrant tenderness. The left femoral pulse is clearly diminished. His legs are mottled."

Silence.

"I think he has a triple-A," I prompted.

"I can't accept him," he said in a dismissive tone. "Only the attending can."

My patient was grimacing. It had to be an aneurysm. Nothing else could account for such pain. I had no more time for dead-end calls.

But I couldn't transfer him yet. Federal laws make it illegal to ship out a patient without an accepting physician and a guaranteed bed on the other end. I called Don, who runs our hospital's ambulance service, and explained the situation.

"You really need this? I'll send one."

An emergency like this doesn't have to happen. Sometimes a doctor can detect an abdominal aortic aneurysm during a routine physical before it leaks and take preventive steps. Many doctors now recommend periodic ultrasounds for high-risk patients. Among people over 65, smokers have four to eight times the average person's risk; those with high blood pressure have double the risk.

A normal abdominal aorta measures 2 centimeters in diameter. When an aneurysm hits 5.5 centimeters, the risk of rupture is 5 to 11 percent. At 6.5 centimeters, the risk more than doubles.

Surgeons can mend the weakened aorta by clamping it, cutting out the ballooned section, and replacing it with a synthetic vessel. Still, this is an operation with a death rate of 2 to 11 percent. Large hospitals with extensive vascular experience give the best odds. It is a soul-searing choice: maybe die now, or probably die later. As a result, many experts recommend holding off on surgery until the aneurysm reaches 6 centimeters or grows more than a centimeter a year or starts causing symptoms.

Researchers are studying a less invasive method. In 1991, surgeons devised a graft that reinforces the aorta from within. First, a catheter is threaded through the groin artery to the level of the aneurysm. Then a sheath on the catheter is pulled back to let the tubular graft spring open and latch onto the vessel's wall with tiny hooks. When all goes according to plan, the new conduit then seals off the aneurysm from the circulation.

If this method works out, the 200,000 patients diagnosed each year could be spared major surgery, and perhaps smaller aneurysms could be repaired sooner. So far, the verdict is good but not definitive. Over a thousand have been inserted, with mortality rates ranging from 0 to 6 percent. One drawback is that many patients do not have the right plumbing for the graft. Their aortas are too heavily calcified or narrowed by blockages to hold the graft. More worrisome is the grafts' tendency to leak blood around their seals. This can occur in up to a third of the cases, often causing the aneurysm to keep expanding. The follow-up time for most of these endovascular grafts has been six to eighteen months, too short to know if there are long-term disasters looming. Moreover, a stampede to the new procedure might make it impossible to enroll patients in a clinical trial that fairly compares it to traditional surgery.

But for our patient, the question was no longer whether, or what, but when.

Just then the ambulance crew arrived.

In a last-ditch attempt at legality, I called the emergency room uptown. By luck, I stumbled on an acquaintance.

"Lauren, I'm not sure," I began, "but I think it's a leaking triple-A. The vascular resident gave me the runaround. I have no CAT scan or ultrasound . . . or accepting physician…"

"I'll deal with the surgeons. Send him."

Five hours later, she called back.

"Infrarenal triple-A," she said without preamble. "They're almost done."

"Whew," I exhaled. "Thanks so much for taking him."

"My pleasure," she replied, "but tell me something. How did you know?"

Tony Dajer is site director of the emergency division at New York Presbyterian Hospital.

Note: This article was written in 2000. Since then, the safety of endovascular repair has been proved. More remarkably, portable ultrasound machines are now ubiquitous in emergency departments—and ER doctors know how to use them.

CHAPTER

25

WHY CAN'T THIS WOMAN BREATHE?

By Tony Dajer

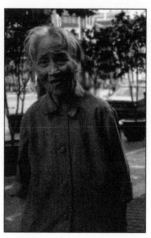

Photo 25-1

The patient was an elderly Chinese immigrant with a history of gastric cancer. She had come into the emergency room in New York City complaining of abdominal pain.

"Tung, tung?" I asked in my laughable Cantonese.

She pinwheeled a hand over her belly. "Pain everywhere."

When I pressed on her abdomen, she grimaced. But she had no fever or evidence of peritonitis, an inflammation of the membrane that lines the abdominal cavity.

"How long?" I asked her English-speaking daughter.

"Two days."

"Getting worse?"

"Yes."

Her abdominal X-rays showed no obstruction. But the X-rays couldn't tell the whole story. Older people can harbor abdominal catastrophes—appendicitis, abscesses, gangrenous gallbladders—without mounting a temperature or yielding the usual physical exam clues.

So, as happens 10 million times a year in this country, I ordered a contrast CT scan—an imaging technique that employs a spinning X-ray beam to take multiple images that create a portrait of internal organs. In a contrast CT scan, additional substances are given to the patient that allow radiologists to better tell one organ from another or detect signs of infection.

First, the patient drinks a quart of what we call an oral contrast—an iodine-based concoction (that comes in a tasty lemon-vanilla flavor) whose high molecular density coats the intestines. Next, we inject six ounces of an intravenous material, also iodinated, to enhance the outline of the blood vessels. These materials weaken the passage of X-rays and make the treated regions appear white against the gray of surrounding tissues. The substances are usually excreted in a few hours.

Sometimes the injected material can be dangerous because of the processing burden it puts on the kidneys. And it can trigger a life-threatening allergic reaction. That occurs some 4,000 times a year in the United States. And what of the oral contrast? Usually, the worst that happens is a little diarrhea. It's about as scary as a milk shake.

The results of the CT scan showed nothing dire. "We will admit you to the hospital," I told her, "and do more tests."

She neither changed her expression nor met my eye.

"The good news is, the tests show nothing seriously wrong," I said.

No reaction.

"How do you feel?"

A slight nod.

"The admitting doctors will be down in a little while."

The daughter formed a thin smile. "Thank you."

An hour later, the patient's nurse, Nina, grabbed me.

"She's bad. She can't breathe. Sounds like airway obstruction."

"Nina, it's her belly, not her lungs."

"You'd better look at her."

I hurried over.

Hrahaahr, hrahaahr came the noise out of her throat. Above the rattle was a high-pitched tone that sounded like stridor, the sound of air being forcibly inhaled through swollen vocal cords or throat membranes. But my patient was making noise as she exhaled. When I listened through the stethoscope, her lungs sounded clear. The trouble was in her throat, but her breathing didn't make sense. A straw is supposed to collapse when you suck on it, not when you blow out.

Nina and I quickly moved her to a fully monitored bed. The pulse oximeter showed the level of blood oxygen to be 90 percent—terrible, no; marginal, yes. I considered the possibilities.

One was an allergic reaction to the scanning material she was given intravenously, which could cause vocal cord and laryngeal tissues to swell. But that would trigger stridor, not this bizarre-sounding exhalation. Another scenario: if the oral scanning material gets into the bronchial tubes that lead into the lungs, it can absorb a large amount of water and clog the airway. But the patient had drunk the concoction hours ago.

The larynx, however, is a bit like a Rube Goldberg contraption. Made up of nine different cartilages, it lies behind the tongue, jutting up like a half-buried, trumpet-shaped pitcher plant. The vocal cords, deep within, stretch from top to bottom. With every swallow, the trapdoor of the epiglottis drops over the opening, shutting off the entrance to the larynx. During the swallow, the whole laryngeal apparatus moves up and forward under the tongue, which, with a powerful back kick, propels the contents of the mouth into the esophagus. It requires split-second coordination of muscle, nerve, and cartilage to catapult food, drink, and saliva over the voice box and into the gullet.

As it happens, a little trough runs between the epiglottis and the tongue, and several pits lie behind the laryngeal opening, where secretions or food particles can accumulate. When we clear our throats, that's generally the stuff we're bringing up. Despite vocal cords that slam shut at the least irritation and a cough reflex that can blast air out at 50 miles an hour, fully half of healthy people inhale some stomach contents during sleep. As we age, weakened muscles and sluggish reflexes aggravate the problem. Every year many thousands of pneumonia cases among older people result from misswallowed food and drink.

I wondered if some of the oral contrast had pooled around my patient's larynx, setting off irritation and swelling. Maybe she had then coughed some up and inhaled it.

Nurses and medical residents stood at her bedside. The level of oxygen in her blood had sagged into the 80s—definitely not good. I leaned over her bed rail to listen closely. The *hrahaahr, hrahaahr* rattled my ribs. Beads of sweat broke out on her face as she fought harder to breathe.

Upper airway obstruction but not stridor? The question raced inside my mind.

As a treatment of last resort we could inject epinephrine, also known as adrenaline, which is the most potent of anti-allergy drugs. But this woman was 75 years old: the adrenaline boost could easily jolt her heart into a lethal rhythm. Besides, she showed no signs of a body-wide allergic reaction. The more I listened, the more obvious it seemed that her problem lay in the throat.

Two surgery residents were passing by. "I may need you here in a minute," I told them. "If we can't turn her around, she could be too swollen to intubate. Might need a trach."

If we couldn't slip a breathing tube down her narrowed throat, we would need to cut a hole in the windpipe, or trachea, to create an airway. A tracheostomy is a bloody and usually panic-lit procedure. We needed to be ready.

"*Hrahaahr, hrahaahr,*" she brayed. Her oxygen level now read 85 percent. We were losing ground.

"Somebody call a doctor," I muttered.

The residents chuckled. They thought I was kidding.

Then I remembered another way to administer epinephrine. When children have croup, a viral infection that causes swelling in the trachea below the vocal cords, we give a different type of epinephrine—called racemic epinephrine—that can be inhaled. The inhaled mist constricts blood vessels in the airway and reduces inflammation. But I'd never used it on an adult.

"Nina, how about some racemic epinephrine?" I said. "You know, the kind we use on croupy kids."

She looked doubtful. "I'll take a look."

"It can't really hurt," I wheedled.

The vials came down. Nina read and reread the instructions. She poured the clear liquid into a pod-shaped container, attached it to a mask, hooked up oxygen delivery, and strapped the contraption around the patient's face. With a sharp hiss, a cloud filled the face mask. She breathed in and out a dozen times.

Precisely 45 seconds later the noise ceased. We all looked at each other. I listened again to her chest. Air, sibilant and clean, whistled through it.

"I'll be darned," I said.

Nina wasn't sure. "Could it act so fast?"

"Oh, epinephrine works fast," I told her. "I'm just surprised it worked at all. Maybe some of the contrast stayed in her throat and made everything swell up, or maybe it gurgled into her airway."

"Hours later?" Nina asked.

"The anatomy ain't perfect, you know."

Ten minutes later, the patient got a little noisy again.

"Let's give her another," I told Nina.

Forty-five seconds later, there was the same result—this time for good.

"You convinced?" I asked Nina.

"Sure. But what's the diagnosis?"

"Beats me," I confessed. "But I'll take a good cure over a clear diagnosis any day."

The woman's belly pain went away on its own over the next two days. In retrospect, she probably hadn't needed the CT scan. But at least there was no more trouble with her airway. My best guess was that the oral material must have been the culprit—and I tried not to wonder how many patients undergo unnecessary CT scans. One thing I was sure of, though: it would be good to always be so lucky.

Tony Dajer is site director of the emergency division at New York Presbyterian Hospital.

THE DISEASE THAT SHOWS US HOW WE ARE WHAT WE EAT

By Tony Dajer

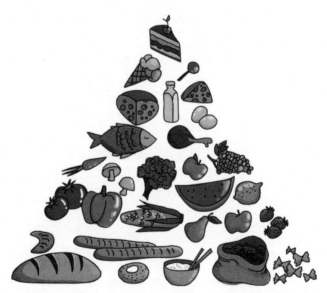

Photo 26-1

A half-dozen people milled uncertainly around a woman on a stretcher. One of them asked, *"A ver, quién la va a atender, que está mala."* (Who will see to her? She is in pain.) They scanned the harshly lit emergency room for someone to trust. The spiky rhythms of their Argentine accents were unmistakable.

"Buenas noches," I said. *"¿Cómo les puedo ayudar?"* (How may I help you?)

"This is my mother, Carmen Beneto," her daughter said, taking the older woman's hand. Beneto, although pale and obviously in pain, inclined her head with understated dignity.

"She has been sick for a week but only just let us know. It wasn't so bad. Until now," she said, smiling ruefully.

Jackie, the triage nurse, took her vital signs. "Temp's 102, pulse 130," she said, giving me her this-one-is-sick look.

We wheeled her into a slot.

"Where are you from?" I asked.

"Buenos Aires."

I examined her. Her lungs were clear: no obvious pneumonia. Her heart was normal. "I've never been. Beautiful?"

"Very," she replied with feeling.

I listened at her abdomen, tapping the tip of my right middle finger against the last knuckle of the left. "How old are you?"

"Seventy."

"Does this hurt?"

"Yes, I must admit it does," she replied, wincing to a very gentle tap.

"Where does it feel the worst?"

"Here, on the left, lower down."

"How long?"

"Well, it began softly, on the plane."

"A week ago?"

"I'm afraid, yes. Sometimes it would retreat a little."

"Any nausea, vomiting?"

"No. I tried to keep eating well. I didn't want to worry anyone."

"What did you do today?"

"Today she walked across the Brooklyn Bridge," her daughter interjected.

By now I was convinced she had a belly full of pus caused by an infection of the intestinal wall. Incredulous, I asked, "The whole way?"

"It is captivating," she said sheepishly.

"What do you do?" I inquired.

"I am a professor of Spanish literature at the University of Buenos Aires," she said.

"Did you know Jorge Luis Borges?" I asked teasingly.

"Of course." She smiled. "What conversations we had together."

"You knew Jorge Luis Borges? Who wrote about libraries that branch off to infinity? Where novels get rewritten in the particle of time it takes a firing-squad bullet to fly?"

"His library would beguile you for a lifetime. And now, my doctor, what diagnostic branches are you exploring?"

"By your exam and symptoms . . . it may be peritonitis."

"Ah," she said thoughtfully, as if presented with a rare ornithological specimen. "I imagine this is serious."

"Yes. It probably stems from a diverticulitis. In the colon."

"You are not sure?"

"Doctors should never be sure too soon. A CT scan will help."

No disease better proves that we are what we eat than diverticulitis. Virtually unheard of before 1900, the condition has emerged as one of the booby prizes of progress. A diverticulum (diverticula is the plural) is a small pouch protruding from the colon—or any hollow organ—that shouldn't be there. Diverticulosis is the condition of having many of these pouches. And diverticulitis is what happens when the pouches get infected.

The rise of the disease in England around World War I has been attributed to changes in the way flour was made some 30 years earlier, when mills began removing two-thirds of the wheat's fiber during processing. Other evidence also supports a link to a lack of dietary fiber. Diverticulitis is nonexistent in rural sub-Saharan Africans, who eat a fiber-rich diet, yet it is common among the city dwellers of Johannesburg. Studies of rats have shown that those fed on a low-fiber diet have five times the incidence of diverticulosis as those fed a roughage-rich diet.

Draped around the abdomen like an inverted U, the colon's main job is to absorb water from liquid stool before it is expelled. How fiber helps keep it healthy is unclear. One possible explanation is that a high-bulk diet expands the colon, whereas a low-bulk diet narrows it. And a narrowed colon must generate higher pressures per square inch to move its contents along. Eventually that pressure may force the colon to bulge out at weak spots, where nourishing blood vessels penetrate the colon wall. Over time, these bulges enlarge into true blind sacs—diverticula. It is no coincidence that most (but not all) diverticula occur in the descending left colon, where forces are greatest.

By themselves, the little sacs are harmless. But the blood vessels alongside them can rupture and bleed. More dangerous still, bacteria-laden stool can leak through the intestinal wall onto the outer surfaces of the intestines, the peritoneum.

Not surprisingly, diverticulosis is most common among the elderly. But it can also occur in young people. I once examined a 24-year-old man complaining of two days' pain in the left lower quadrant of his abdomen. He had had no fever, nausea, vomiting, or diarrhea—in short, no symptoms of an intestinal disorder. I decided he had pulled an abdominal muscle and sent him home. The next day another doctor sent him to a surgeon, who to my dismay found a large diverticular abscess.

Diverticulitis is deceptive and insidious. About a fifth of diverticulosis sufferers will, on occasion, complain of abdominal pain and a change in bowel function. The challenge for doctors is to identify those who harbor a true infection. The process begins when a weakened sac bursts, spilling feces into the abdominal cavity. Even then, fever and an elevated white blood cell count may be absent for days. Pain may be vague and hard to localize, or may arise deceptively on the right. Luckily, the body can often wall off the leaking bacteria and suppress infection. But if one ignores the early symptoms, and the spillage is either large or spreads quickly, the result can be a deep-seated abscess, peritonitis, or both.

"*Profesora* Beneto," I said, holding up the film of her CT scan, "there appears to be an abscess. Here, where the left colon begins its descent to the rectum."

The professor and her daughter studied the white-on-black images. The circle with the moth-eaten interior—the diverticular abscess—was unmistakable. Gravely, she asked, "I suppose this will not resolve with antibiotics alone?"

I shook my head.

"Does that mean the artificial rectum? And the bag?"

"Very likely, I am afraid. But it will not be permanent. In several months the colon can be reconnected."

"There is no other way?"

I said nothing. She understood.

Less dire cases of diverticulitis can often be cured with oral antibiotics and a liquid diet, which relieves the pressures on the colon. Moreover, some abscesses can frequently be drained by using a CT scan to determine where to slip the needle through the skin or rectum. But for my stoic professor, it was too late. There was too much pus and too much inflammation. Peritonitis, even treated with latest-generation antibiotics, can kill a healthy 30 year old. And although cutting out a segment of the colon and reattaching the ends is technically easy, the repair could get badly infected and spill more bacteria-rich stool. The safest course is to perform a colostomy: Excise the infected portion of colon, then create an artificial exit for the upper colon that remains. The resulting portal looks a bit like a fish's mouth emerging from the water.

When the surgeons cut into Professora Beneto's abdomen, foul-smelling, greenish-yellow pus oozed out. To cleanse the infected area, they repeatedly poured saline into the abdominal cavity and suctioned it away. After draining the abscess, they removed about three feet of colon, then created the artificial opening. Throughout the operation, Professor Beneto's vital signs stayed rock-stable.

"Like a 20 year old's," one of the surgeons told me later.

Four days later, I visited the professor. She was sitting up, sipping fluids, surrounded by her family. She would not return to solid foods until well after her colon had healed.

"Ah, Doctor," she said, lifting a hand in greeting, "What do you think Jorge Luis would remark on this business of seeing one's insides on the outside?"

"He would say beautiful bridges can indeed nurture the soul," I replied. "But he might add that the body sometimes needs to get itself to the doctor."

Tony Dajer is site director of the emergency division at New York Presbyterian Hospital.

CHAPTER

27

THE BLOOD PRESSURE MYSTERY

By Tony Dajer

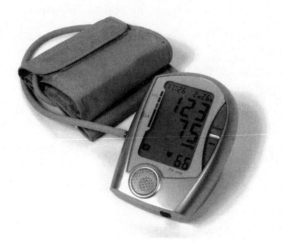

Photo 27-1

I peeked into the emergency room cubicle as our nurse manager filled me in. "Fifty-two-year-old. Sudden nausea and weakness. Blood pressure's low: 66 over 40. Only history is obesity surgery four years ago." Vincent, my fellow attending, stood at the bedside. Mr. Dexter, the patient, was alert and uncomplaining.

"Can't be too sick. Probably vasovagal," I thought, walking on. The vasovagal reaction is a catchall term for a transient condition involving fear or pain, such as gastrointestinal upset, that causes low blood pressure, slow heart rate, and in some cases fainting. Patients who have had gastric bypass surgery, a treatment for obesity that dramatically reduces the size of the stomach, often experience such upset. The condition usually passes quickly.

An hour later, Vincent buttonholed me. "Could you help me look at his heart?" he asked. "We've given three liters of saline, plus dopamine [a blood pressure booster]. Blood pressure won't come up. EKG shows no heart attack. No fever, headache, chest pain, or abdominal pain," he added. "Maybe the ventricle wall isn't contracting right. EKGs don't always pick up heart attacks."

The numbers on the monitor jolted me: still 66 over 40. So much for my snap diagnosis.

I wheeled the ultrasound machine over.

"What does that do, Doctor?"

"We're going to look at your heart," I told Mr. Dexter. "No chest pain, right?"

"That's correct, Doctor."

"Tell me again what happened."

"I was sitting at my desk," he related. "A wave of weakness hit me, then I got short of breath. Nausea, too."

"No pain anywhere?"

"Not that I can recall."

His heart looked fine. He didn't have fever, vomiting, or diarrhea.

In medical parlance, a drop in blood pressure is known as shock. It has nothing to do with emotional upset and everything to do with hydraulics. When blood pressure suddenly dips, there are three main possible causes: pump failure (as in a heart attack), leaky blood vessels (an immune response to an overwhelming infection), or fluid loss (bleeding or dehydration). A systolic pressure of 66 meant Mr. Dexter had lost about two quarts of blood. So where was it? The GI tract—the most common source of spontaneous hemorrhage—was clean.

I placed the ultrasound probe on Mr. Dexter's right flank, where the kidney and liver meet. Anatomists call this spot Morison's pouch. Luckily for emergency room doctors, it's easy to find and happens to be where free fluid in the abdomen accumulates. Immediately a broad black stripe showed up between the grayish-looking liver and the right kidney.

"Lots of free fluid in there," I announced. An ultrasound cannot distinguish between blood and other fluids, but there was no reason for Mr. Dexter to have ascites, the accumulation of fluid in the belly that can come with cirrhosis of the liver.

"Do you have any belly pain?"

"You guys keep asking me that."

"How about this?" I gently pressed a hand into his stomach.

"Okay, okay, that hurts some, but not bad."

Blood can be highly irritating to the abdomen's lining, so if the excess fluid was blood, Mr. Dexter should have felt more pain, but following gastric bypass surgery, he no longer had a normal abdomen.

With low blood pressure and possible blood in the belly, this patient was now an official emergency. "Call the surgeons—now!" I ordered. "Make sure he's typed and crossed for four units." More nurses swarmed in.

An intern entered, waving a slip of paper: "His hematocrit is 26." That's a low—but not critically low—red blood cell count.

"I've been a little anemic in the years since the surgery," Mr. Dexter offered.

"What's your usual level?" I asked.

"Don't know. Sorry."

Don, one of our surgeons, came charging down with his team. "Odd thing is," I told him, "his belly's not tender, but look at this." I passed the ultrasound wand over the black band again.

"I see it," Don said. "I believe you."

"Could he have a PE?" the chief surgical resident mused, referring to a pulmonary embolus, or blood clot in the lung. "The gastric bypass puts him at risk. Or maybe a suture line eroded or there's a perforation leaking stomach contents."

The list of possibilities seemed endless. With no time to spare and Mr. Dexter too unstable to undergo a CT scan to image the lung, we would have to decide on an operation based on our own judgment.

"Why should a healthy man suddenly bleed into his belly?" Don asked. "And then not be tender? What if it's a PE and we operate, then have to anticoagulate him? Nightmare."

"His oxygen level's not bad," I said.

"It's like he has half of everything," the chief resident observed.

"How about we look at his heart with a bedside echocardiogram?" I suggested. "If the pulmonary artery is corked by a clot, we'll see a dilated right ventricle." Echocardiograms create images of a beating heart, to help doctors spot problems in cardiac structure and function. Mr. Dexter's results were normal.

"We've wasted enough time. Let's go," Don ordered.

Suddenly the monitor beeped: Blood pressure was now 110 over 60. Mr. Dexter was in safer territory now.

I held Don back. "His blood pressure's better. Maybe something clotted off. Why don't we sneak a CT scan on the way up?"

Fifteen minutes later, everyone crowded into the radiology suite. The scan showed blood everywhere.

"What's that?" Don tapped the lower pole of the spleen, where an odd lesion that resembled a bull's-eye lay at the center of the bleeding. "Aneurysm? Tumor?"

"I don't know," the radiologist replied. "Never seen anything like it."

"Guess there's only one way to find out," Don concluded.

What we saw suggested an aneurysm—a malformation of a blood vessel, an uncommon but devilish ailment. Most stem from genetically influenced defects in proteins of the arterial wall. Aneurysms, which bulge like a balloon squeezed too tightly, often arise at an artery's branching point, though they can pop up anywhere. Until they burst without warning, they can escape diagnosis because the irritation caused by blood mimics that of a common infection or even a migraine. In adults 30 to 60 years old, aneurysms rupture most frequently in the brain, causing tens of thousands of fatal or disabling hemorrhages each year. Women are particularly vulnerable. The abdominal aorta, for its part, can bulge out and burst anywhere, but only rarely does this happen in someone under 55.

Then there are the odd ducks, like splenic artery aneurysms. The spleen lies under the left diaphragm, behind the ninth, tenth, and eleventh ribs. It's like the body's oil filter, trapping old red blood cells and certain types of bacteria and removing them from circulation. Unfortunately, the spleen's good-size artery is at risk for an aneurysm during pregnancy, particularly in the third trimester, when the enlarging uterus presses on the vessel, increasing its blood pressure. I know of four cases of ruptured splenic artery aneurysms in pregnant women, each presenting as upper-abdominal pain and vomiting in the third trimester. Flummoxed doctors mistook them for stomach viruses—until the patients' blood pressure plummeted. Two of the women died; the others were saved by last-minute surgery.

Don't fret too much about your plumbing, though. We *Homo sapiens* are well-put-together organisms. Blowing a gasket is a rare event. However, given that the body will do everything possible to keep blood pressure up, a sudden drop should, in this age of bedside ultrasound, prompt a quick look at the plumbing. There is no easier way to save a life.

Three hours later, Don swung by the emergency room, digital camera in hand. "It was a bulge, like an aneurysm, where the artery enters the spleen," he told me, clicking through photos of the crescent-shaped maroon organ. "Splenic peliosis. Ridiculously rare. Cause unknown. Good thing we had the CT scan. Getting through all the adhesions from the gastric bypass surgery was tough, but at least we knew where to go. Luckily for him, it had partly clotted.

"Oh, and you know why the belly wasn't tender?" he continued. "Adhesions from the gastric bypass had stuck his intestines up against the abdominal wall, forcing the blood to the sides. So even with a belly full of blood, it seemed like a benign exam."

"Whew," I whistled. "Close one."

Two days later, Mr. Dexter was holding court in the intensive care unit. "So, should I play the lottery, Doctor? They tell me I'm a million-to-one shot," he joked. He looked so healthy I wanted to click my heels.

"No need for that. We already won," I told him. "You are the jackpot."

Tony Dajer is site director of the emergency division at New York Presbyterian Hospital.

CHAPTER

28

MARY GROVE WAS SUDDENLY SHEDDING SKIN IN LARGE RED PATCHES. THE LOSS WAS A THREAT TO HER LIFE.

By Robert A. Norman

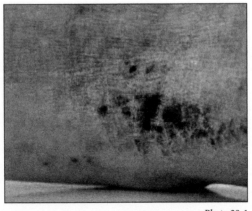

Photo 28-1

My friend Bill Cook, a primary care physician, called me one morning. "I've admitted a patient, a 28-year-old woman," he said. "She's losing her skin. Can you come and take a look at her?" He explained that the patient, Mary Grove, had come to his office the day before, complaining that her skin had suddenly begun to peel. She felt strange—weak and tender—and her eyes and mouth felt irritated. I am a dermatologist, and from Bill's description, I had a good idea of what was wrong with Mary.

Before going in to see her, I reviewed her chart. Mary worked as a receptionist and had a husband and two small children. She had felt fine until the day she was hospitalized. The hospital staff performed routine tests, including a chest X-ray and blood tests. They also put Mary on intravenous fluid replacement therapy and pain medications.

I found Mary in her bed, staring at the flickering images on the TV. When I introduced myself she smiled and said, "Hey."

"I'd like to take a look at your skin," I said, "if that's okay."

"What's left of it," she offered.

With the help of a nurse, I began the exam. We both donned gloves and the nurse gently pulled back the bedsheet. I tried to remain expressionless. Mary was looking right at me, and I didn't want to panic her. Her skin was a blanket of red. The top layer was sloughing off her face, neck, trunk, legs, and feet in large sheets like wet wallpaper. Scattered over her body were a few islands of normal-looking skin. I had seen two other patients with this disorder, but neither of this severity. To determine the extent of the damage, I took a look at the mucous membranes of her mouth, genitals, and eyes.

"Whaddaya think, Doctor?" she slurred. Apparently, she was groggy from her pain medications.

"It appears that you've had a fairly severe reaction to a medicine you took," I said. "It doesn't happen very often, but when it does, it can be a real challenge to care for. But we're going to make sure you get the care you need to recover. It will take some time, but we'll try to make you as comfortable as possible."

"Do you know what happened to me?"

"I have a pretty good idea. But can you answer a few questions first? Have you taken any medicines in the last few weeks?"

"I take something for my knees. It's like a pain pill, but it never gave me a problem before."

"Anything else?"

She paused, her eyes focusing somewhere on the ground. "I did have an earache and I took something I found in my cabinet. I'd have to check it. I remember one of the kids or somebody used it when they had an infection and it helped, so I took it for a few days."

"How long ago did you take it?" I asked.

"I think it was about two weeks ago," she said.

"And this just started a day or two ago?" I asked.

"Day before yesterday, yeah, I started losing my skin. Felt hot all over and sick to my stomach. First I just had the rash on my face, arms, and legs, and then it was all over, even my lips and my eyes. I got these blisters like I was in one of those horror movies after a nuclear explosion."

"Can you have the medicine brought here?" I asked.

"Sure," she said.

"Are you in much pain?" I asked.

"Not really. I feel kind of stoned," she said. "But I'm trying to take in everything you're telling me."

"The pain medications can make you feel quite tired," I said.

Do you remember the last time you had a minor burn? Do you remember how a small part of your skin peeled off? The same reaction extended all across Mary's body. Imagine her the day before her skin erupted: brushing her hair, putting on her makeup, touching herself with a dab of perfume, rubbing moisturizer on her supple, fully intact skin. Put yourself in her busy life, working and taking care of her family. Now here she was, immobilized, her skin peeling off, in the company of hospital monitors and buzzers. But Mary's injury hadn't been caused by anything external, like a burn. The mutiny arose from within.

I explained to Mary that she was probably suffering an extreme and unusual allergic reaction to one of the drugs she had taken. Her immune system, for unknown reasons, viewed it as an enemy and initiated a defense against it. The reaction—called toxic epidermal necrolysis, or TEN—is poorly understood, but the devastation of the skin resembles burn injuries.

"We need to watch you very carefully over the next several days to make sure you don't get an infection or lose too much of your vital fluids," I explained. "The skin acts as a barrier to bacteria; therefore we have to take every precaution to protect you until your skin returns in full. And we'll need to make sure you get enough fluids. The skin is like a regulator to help make sure the right amount of fluid stays in and the correct amount goes out. Without skin, you lose the principal way your body maintains fluid balance."

I paused, giving her time to absorb my little speech. "It looks as though you've lost most of your skin surface, and it will take some time to build a new one. You need the IV fluids so you don't become dehydrated. And we have to be very careful about infection. Please be patient and hang on."

"Okay, Doctor," she said.

"I'll need to send a small sample of your skin to the pathologist. It will help in confirming your diagnosis."

"Whatever. It's okay," Mary said. "I probably won't feel it too much."

Mary was right; she showed very little discomfort as I anesthetized the irritated skin and used a tiny punch tool to extract a sample from her left thigh. I put it into the biopsy bottle and sent it off to the pathologist for analysis.

I explained to Mary's nurse the care she would need, then called Bill Cook to put together a treatment plan. We would stabilize her in the internal medicine unit of our hospital and then closely monitor her condition.

On the second day of her hospitalization, I got back the pathologist's report, which confirmed my diagnosis. On the third day of hospitalization, we moved Mary to the burn unit, where the staff is trained to care for patients with severe skin loss. They carefully removed the dead skin and applied a loose gauze dressing saturated with antibacterial agents to the denuded skin surface. The staff made sure she was getting enough fluids and nutrients and carefully monitored her fluid intake and urine output. They also kept a close watch on her general condition and vital signs—pulse, respiration, temperature. They monitored her blood for signs of infection or irregularities relating to fluid loss. And each half hour they checked the blood pressure near her heart, which would reveal the first signs of fluid imbalance.

I also called in an ophthalmologist to check Mary's eyes. She had complained that they were dry, and eye damage is common among TEN patients.

Mary was one of about 500 cases of toxic epidermal necrolysis in the United States each year. Although the disorder is considered rare, its frequency may be underestimated because mild cases probably go unreported. Most reported cases, like Mary's, pop up one to three weeks after a new drug is taken. The onset is rapid and in some cases can be terribly severe. Patients can lose their entire epidermis—the uppermost of the skin's three layers—within about 24 hours.

The greatest threat to patients with toxic epidermal necrolysis is not the damage to the skin itself but the manner in which that damage increases a patient's vulnerability to infection. When the epidermis is destroyed, the body surface is a standing invitation to pathogens. Destroyed skin tissue is an excellent environment for bacteria, and within a very short time bacteria contaminating the injury begin to multiply. If left untreated, the infection can spread—with disastrous consequences. Roughly 30 percent of patients diagnosed with TEN die—most often because infection has spread into their bloodstreams.

The usual treatment is a topical antimicrobial agent. But first the dead skin must be carefully removed and the area cleansed to speed recovery. Then the denuded area is covered with antimicrobial ointment and a sterile dressing. Applying ice or cold water can help reduce pain and decrease injury. A tetanus shot is also given; this is standard in patients with open wounds who, like Mary, have no recent record of immunization.

The inflammatory reaction is not limited to the skin. The mucous membranes of the eyes, mouth, genitals, and anus often show redness and widespread tissue destruction. Patients can shed the epidermis of the eyelids, as well as eyebrows, fingernails, and toenails. In severe cases the inflammation can extend to the internal organs, causing damage to the intestinal and respiratory tracts. Mary was, in this respect, fortunate. Her internal symptoms were limited to some inflammation in her mouth. A topical ointment helped heal and anesthetize the tender inflamed sites.

Most patients suffer damage only in the epidermis. Blood vessels in the dermis—the layer of skin beneath the epidermis—may swell but remain intact. Within a month, the skin heals, although some residual redness may linger for a few weeks. In some extremely severe cases the damage may extend past the dermis to the subcutaneous layer of skin. When patients suffer this much destruction—which is as severe as a third-degree burn—they need skin grafts.

The prognosis for TEN depends on how quickly the disorder is diagnosed and treated. The peak of the disease (by the third day, in Mary's case) bears the highest threat, and the fate of the patient often hangs in the balance for one or more weeks. Nearly half of the surviving patients have residual and potentially disabling eye lesions, which can include scarring of the cornea. Mary's chances for recovery were good, given that we identified and treated the disorder quickly.

What brings about this terrible eruption? The underlying cause is probably an overactive immune response. But until we understand what sparks the deranged immune reaction, there is no way to prevent it. Fortunately, our methods for treating the injury and preventing devastating infection have improved over the past few years.

What we do know about TEN is that drugs are the most common culprit. But most cases involve patients on several drugs, so it can be difficult to pinpoint the offending medication. Mary, unlike most TEN patients, had taken only one new drug—a medication for ear pain containing sulfa, which probably ignited the eruption.

After a week in the hospital Mary improved, and within a month she was up and around. Her eyes appeared to have been spared any chronic harm. When I saw Mary just before she was discharged from the hospital, I gave her a list of medicines containing sulfa that she had to avoid. She was in no way, I emphasized, immune to a recurrence. In fact, she continues to be at high risk for TEN if she ever takes products containing sulfa.

I saw Mary for a follow-up visit about a month later. She had fared well. Most of her skin had healed nicely. She said her eye doctor thought her right cornea was a little damaged, but her eyesight had not been harmed. Amazingly, Mary had emerged more or less unscathed. She bore only a slight visible trace of the vast tissue destruction: a small spot of scar tissue on her left thigh.

Robert A. Norman is a dermatologist in Tampa, Florida, and the author of The Woman Who Lost Her Skin and Other Dermatological Tales.

CHAPTER
29

BENIGN BUT IRRITATING SKIN ERUPTIONS SIGNAL MUCH MORE SERIOUS INTERNAL TROUBLES

By Robert A. Norman

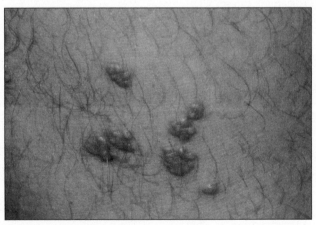

Photo 29-1

As a dermatologist, I see many skin disorders but rarely anything so revealing—and misleading—at the same time.

"There are lots of bumps coming up," my new patient told me.

Dozens of tiny yellow and pinkish eruptions ringed in red were scattered over his chest, abdomen, upper and lower extremities, and back.

"How long has this been happening?" I asked.

"Three months. I went to the walk-in clinic, and the doctor said to come see you."

"Did they do any tests?"

When a person has problems metabolizing cholesterol and triglycerides, those substances may accumulate in patches on the skin called xanthomas. The pinkish or yellow patches consist not only of extracellular lipids but also scavenging immune cells.

"Nope."

"Do these bumps bother you?" I asked.

"Sometimes. Kind of itchy."

"Do you remember if they came on gradually or suddenly?"

"It was like all at once. One day they just seemed to be there."

I checked his chart: 37 years old. He had a hernia repair as a child and a history of unspecified back surgery. Now he had hypertension and occasional abdominal pain. He was taking medications for pain, depression, and high blood pressure.

"Any particular diseases run in the family?" I asked.

"I was adopted when I was 2. I don't know anything about my natural parents or family."

"What about your diet?"

"Not real great lately."

"Such as?"

"I eat about three gallons of ice cream and a bottle of chocolate syrup every week."

I noted this on his chart but said nothing. Doctors are trained not to be judgmental. He was 5-foot-8 and weighed 230 pounds. His blood pressure was 142 over 88, and his pulse was 92. He had checked off "yes" to smoking—one and a half packs of tobacco a day for approximately twenty years—and occasional alcohol use. He said he didn't use illicit drugs.

For more clues, I shaved a bit of the skin eruption for analysis, and I ordered tests of his fasting lipid profile, complete blood count, and blood chemistry.

"What the heck is going on with me?" he asked.

"The growths are not any kind of cancer, but they could be a sign of a problem inside. You need to get the laboratory tests done as soon as possible. And I'll be seeing you right after that."

Before he left I made sure he was scheduled again for an appointment and dictated a letter to the doctor he'd seen at the walk-in clinic.

A few days later, the biopsy result confirmed my suspicions: eruptive xanthoma, a type of benign skin growth made up of macrophages (immune cells) filled with fatty substances called lipids. Xanthomas are associated with a condition in which lipids—specifically, a type of fat called a triglyceride—accumulate in the blood and elsewhere.

His lab tests showed that his total cholesterol was almost 1,000 and his triglycerides close to 4,000, both dangerously high. His glucose was elevated at over 200, and his liver enzymes—an indication of systemic problems that can accompany xanthomas— were also up. I left a message on his answering machine to contact me right away. About two hours later, I got a call from his father.

"You're the dermatologist, right?"

"Yes," I said.

"He had good things to say about you. I talked to him about you just yesterday."

"How is he doing?"

"Not so good. He's in the hospital with a heart attack. Got up this morning and complained of chest pain that kept getting worse. Luckily I was here to rush him over there."

His father told me where he was and who was treating him.

"I appreciate your calling me," I said. "Sorry he's in bad shape."

I arranged to have the patient's recent blood and biopsy reports along with my contact information faxed to the hospital.

Later, the attending doctor called. "I'm glad you sent us your findings," he said. "Your reports saved us a lot of time and helped us get his treatment going in the right direction." He went on to explain that they found severe premature atherosclerosis and an enlarged left ventricle. "We're getting some more specific tests," he added. "He should be out of the ICU in a couple of days if all goes well. If we keep him alive, he'll be rooming with us for a while."

"I'm sure it'll take time. But I have a question. I have seen others with this problem, and they've had pancreatitis. What's different here?"

"This guy was playing with fire," the attending doctor said.

"How's that?" I asked.

"We do routine toxicity tests, and he came back positive for cocaine. High levels. So on top of this lipid problem he was pushing his heart even harder."

Many conditions that perturb lipid metabolism can cause xanthomas, including diabetes, low thyroid, and alcohol abuse, and in women, the use of estrogen. But the doctor suspected a different explanation: Cocaine use had heightened a preexisting genetic vulnerability to heart problems.

The patient's prematurely narrowed arteries and high lipid levels were strong clues. A variety of protein defects can disrupt normal function and cause lipids to accumulate in the blood, infiltrate the walls of blood vessels, and form deposits on the skin. The conditions are often inherited, and patients typically develop atherosclerosis in their twenties or thirties. Skin eruptions are a common symptom. The patient didn't know his biological family's medical vulnerabilities because he had been adopted.

In someone whose arteries are already prematurely narrowed, cocaine use will make a heart attack even more likely. Cocaine damages the heart by triggering the release of epinephrine and norepinephrine, hormones that cause arteries to constrict, force the heart to work harder, and sometimes induce a spasm in the coronary arteries. Cocaine also damages the heart wall itself, although why this occurs is not well understood. The relationship of cocaine use to heart problems was first documented in the early 1970s, and cardiovascular symptoms are now recognized as the most common indicator of cocaine abuse.

Although chronic cocaine use could have provoked accelerated atherosclerosis, the patient's high levels of cholesterol and triglycerides had put a tremendous strain on his cardiovascular system. His tobacco habit had further heightened his risk because cigarette smoke is believed to provoke inflammation in the circulatory system.

A genetic test subsequently confirmed that he had familial dysbetalipoproteinemia, a condition that occurs in about 1 in 10,000 people. While he was hospitalized, the patient began taking a lipid-lowering drug. By interfering with the body's ability to make triglycerides, it would help diminish his cardiac problems and prevent pancreatitis.

I saw him again when he got out of the hospital a month later. His plasma triglyceride levels had fallen to less than 1,000 milligrams per deciliter, and the xanthomas were beginning to disappear.

He looked a bit more relaxed than during his first office visit. "I appreciate your getting those blood tests and a skin sample. The doctor in the hospital told me that helped save me."

We talked about his drug use, his genetic vulnerability, and how the xanthomas developed.

"I cleaned up my act," he said.

"If you can be honest with yourself, it helps," I said. "And be truthful to your health care providers. You almost lost your life." If he used cocaine again, I explained, it would be like a time bomb set to go off.

"I ain't no terrorist," he said. "Especially against myself."

I saw him about six months later. This time, his blood fats were getting back to normal levels, and the xanthomas had almost vanished. He had confronted an unknown genetic legacy and a self-destructive drug habit, and he was lucky to be alive.

Robert A. Norman is a dermatologist in Tampa, Florida, and the author of The Woman Who Lost Her Skin and Other Dermatological Tales.

CHAPTER

30

A SONG FROM *SHREK* HELPS A 5-YEAR-OLD BOY RECOVER FROM DIFFICULT SURGERY

By Burak Ozgur

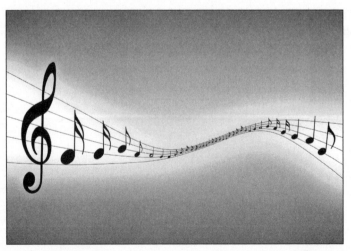

Photo 30-1

One afternoon in late June, I was called to the emergency room to look over a CT scan of the brain of a young boy. The 5 year old's troubles had begun a while back with headaches and vision problems. After visits to his pediatrician and an ophthalmologist, he got a prescription for new glasses. The family thought the matter was solved.

Several months later, though, the child's mother noticed that he had difficulty with balance. Then he developed early-morning headaches with nausea and vomiting. The boy's pediatrician told his parents that he must be evaluated immediately, so they brought him to the emergency room of the Children's Hospital in San Diego, where I am a resident in neurosurgery.

The CT scan showed dilation of the ventricles, the fluid-filled cavities in the brain. This expansion is almost always caused by a blockage, and a detailed MRI soon found the source: a tumor in a region of the brain known as the posterior fossa. This area includes the cerebellum, the part of the brain known for its role in balance and coordination.

The posterior fossa also includes the fourth ventricle, one of the main pathways through which cerebrospinal fluid, the liquid that bathes and cushions the brain, travels down to the spinal cord. If the pathway gets blocked, the fluid accumulates and presses on the brain. The pressure can cause different effects depending on what spot is being compressed. One result can be headaches and vomiting.

Unfortunately, the MRI could not tell us what kind of tumor we had found. But I knew that two types of pediatric tumors commonly occur in this part of the brain. The first is pilocytic astrocytoma, which develops when a type of supportive, non-neuronal brain cell called an astrocyte grows out of control. This type of tumor tends to develop as a nodule that is usually easy to remove.

The second is a medulloblastoma, a cancer that is thought to develop from embryonic cells that persist in the brain. Medulloblastomas are more difficult to treat—and remove— than pilocytic astrocytomas are because they tend to grow in a mass that infiltrates surrounding brain tissue. We would not know which one the boy had without taking it out and analyzing it. Michael Levy, the hospital's chief of pediatric neurosurgery, and Hal Meltzer, an attending pediatric neurosurgeon, would be participating in the surgery and treatment, which was scheduled for the next morning.

We began by drilling into the skull to insert a tube into the fluid-filled cavities so we could drain the accumulated cerebrospinal fluid and relieve the pressure. Then we cut away a small piece of the skull to get at the round, walnut-size tumor. The brain tissue below was pinkish orange, and the borders of the growth were clearly visible. We carefully excised the tumor, replaced the portion of skull we had removed, and secured it in place with screwed-in titanium plates. The operation took five hours. We left the draining tube in place to reduce pressure on the brain.

The boy's tumor was a medulloblastoma, which carries a greater risk of recurrence or spread of the cancer to other parts of the body than pilocytic astrocytoma. Assuming he recovered from the operation, he would still have to endure chemotherapy, radiation, and continued monitoring for recurrences. He was facing a long recovery.

Following the surgery, he seemed fine. He could move and gesture. He could comprehend others. But he couldn't speak. As the days passed, his situation did not improve.

Unfortunately, the boy had fallen victim to a poorly understood post-operative complication of posterior fossa surgery known as cerebellar mutism. His loss of speech was puzzling because the cerebellum, located at the base of the brain, is known for equilibrium—not speech production. The centers of speech production and comprehension are located in two separate regions of the cerebrum, the upper portion of the brain. These regions were first identified when researchers observed how injuries or strokes in specific parts of the brain were linked to the loss of particular functions. Sophisticated imaging of brain activity has also helped confirm the role of these regions in talking and listening.

Still, the boy's loss of speech wasn't completely unexpected. There have been clues that the cerebellum plays some as yet undefined role in speech. The first description of cerebellar mutism came in 1917, when World War I soldiers who suffered gunshot wounds to the cerebellum were described as having various forms of speech disorders. However, the term cerebellar mutism wasn't coined until 1985. Since then about 200 cases have been reported. This mutism may result from a disruption of the nerves that coordinate muscles of the face and tongue, and most patients regain speech within a few weeks or months.

Over the next few weeks, I developed a close bond with the boy and his family. When his parents and 10-year-old sister visited, I would see how supportive they were and how careful they were to communicate with him by asking only yes-or-no questions he could answer with a nod. Much of the time was spent watching DVDs together. Day in and day out, I visited the child in the pediatric ward and prayed for a break in his odd prison of verbal silence.

Then one day, it seemed, this prayer was answered.

As I walked into his hospital room one day, I saw that his sister had put on a DVD of *Shrek*. As soon as the song "I'm a Believer" came on, the child began to sing along. Everyone in the room was astonished. We played the song over and over again, and each time he managed to get out some of the lyrics. The episode seemed to catalyze his recovery. He was soon producing words with the help of music. Within a few weeks he could once again speak normally.

How had this happened? After searching through some old texts as well as reviewing some more recent case reports, I understood that there are different pathways for different aspects of speech. For example, some stroke patients lose the ability to speak normally, but their ability to speak in song remains intact. Although some researchers had reported that the cerebellum's relevance to speech involves the control of nerves in the oral and facial musculature that produces words, it may also be involved in somehow triggering speech. Maybe one way that can happen is through melody.

Researchers have discovered several examples of multiple or redundant pathways for the same brain function. Some believe that the multiple pathways act as a backup system to protect certain functions in case of injury. But we have only just begun to scratch the surface in understanding the complexities of the brain. What we may perceive today in our limited mortal understanding as redundant or parallel may prove to be a unique function once we understand what is going on. It is through patients like this young boy and appreciating phenomena like these that we may continue to advance in our understanding.

Within a year, the boy returned to school, and he has continued to do remarkably well. His latest MRI shows no sign of recurrence or spread of the cancer. Three years have passed since we met, and I recently visited him and his family. He is doing well in school, at home, and in baseball. After his extraordinary experience, I was glad to see him enjoying all the ordinary pleasures of childhood.

Burak Ozgur is a resident at the University of California San Diego Medical Center.

CHAPTER

31

PRESENT TENSE

By Bruce H. Dobkin

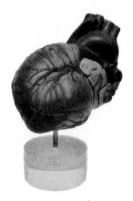

Photo 31-1

His heart surgeons and cardiologist had asked me to clear George for coronary bypass surgery. I had reluctantly given the go-ahead. The atherosclerotic plugs in his coronary arteries had already led to a serious heart attack and a life-threatening irregularity in his heartbeat. George was only 52, a working engineer, the father of two boys in high school. Other therapies had failed. Without surgery he would likely die. How could I recommend withholding a treatment, one that could save his life, simply to avoid the real, but small, chance that he'd suffer a stroke during the operation?

The stroke risk had been higher for George than the usual complication rate of 2 percent because atherosclerosis had partially plugged his basilar artery, the major supplier of blood to the vital centers deep in the brain that control breathing and consciousness. Two of the artery's branches also feed the brain's occipital lobes, which are essential for vision, and two others nurture the inner temporal lobes, which are crucial for remembering new experiences and acquiring new knowledge. Four times in the previous two years, George had endured frightening symptoms for 30 to 90 minutes that had resulted from the narrowing in this artery. He would feel dizzy, lose his balance along with strength in his left arm and leg, go numb in his cheek, see double, slur his speech, and appear confused. Twice he remembered almost nothing about the spells. These transient ischemic attacks, as they're called, were evidence that many of the brain structures fed by the basilar artery were, at least briefly, not getting the blood flow needed to nurture them.

What, then, might happen during coronary bypass surgery, when the heart is temporarily quiescent? Although a mechanical pump usually keeps the blood pressure high enough to perfuse the brain and other organs, the pressure is much lower than usual. When atherosclerosis already narrows the basilar artery, there's a danger that blood flow can become so restricted that some or all of the brain tissue fed by that vessel is destroyed.

George and his wife understood the risk when they agreed to the surgery. That was about a year ago. All had gone well during the operation, until the surgeons took him off the mechanical pump and tried to get his heart beating again. It barely contracted. He was in shock. They put a sausage-shaped balloon into the aorta, the wide artery that leads out from the heart, and rhythmically inflated and collapsed it to mechanically pump blood to his organs. He remained comatose on a respirator. No matter what emergency therapy the team of doctors tried, nothing could get his heart to squeeze powerfully. I stood at the end of his bed in the intensive care unit six hours after the bypass. A dozen flexible tubes penetrated George's body. Fluids of every sort dripped into and out of natural and man-made orifices. His face, chest, and limbs were pale and puffy under the tape that held the maze of tubes and his life together. It was a disaster, a nightmare for his doctors and family. Despite the balloon's pulsations, his entire brain might not be getting the blood supply it needed to protect its billions of cells. More likely, we feared, his vacillating blood pressure between pulsations was often too low to push blood through the basilar artery.

By the next morning, more than one doctor wondered aloud whether we should remove him from the life-sustaining fluids, drugs, and balloon. I could only say that he was not yet brain dead. We had to keep him on life support. I tried to comfort his family, but I worried that George would be left in a vegetative state, like another Karen Ann Quinlan.

Then, nearly two days after surgery, his heart muscle miraculously came alive and pumped vigorously on its own. The surgeons pulled out the balloon. But what would we be left with? He was still in a deep coma when I transferred his neurologic care to an associate for the weekend.

On Monday morning I was astonished to find George moving his arms and legs as he lay in bed wide awake. The tube that connected his trachea to the ventilator prevented him from speaking, but he was able to follow my directions to hold up two fingers, salute, and draw a circle within a square in space. He nodded his head to pick the correct choice for the month and year. His strength, feeling, and coordination tested normal. Tears ran down his wife's face. Somehow, his brain had protected itself. We had not done George in. Two days later, he was out of intensive care.

As I entered his room on my first visit after the last tubes had been removed, he pushed aside the newspaper he was reading, greeted me by name, stood up from his hospital bed, and reached for my hand, as if the ordeal had left no mark. A half-slice of toast and an emptied cereal box lay on his breakfast tray. It was remarkable how good he looked, considering that less than a week had elapsed since the disaster following his surgery. I asked if he had any pain from the chest incision. He said his chest felt sore, but he'd probably lifted something and strained the muscles. It was an odd answer, one that I almost ignored.

I noticed a coat and silk scarf thrown over a nearby chair. "Has your wife already been in to see you?" I asked.

"I think she'll be here soon," George replied.

"You don't recall seeing her this morning?" I reiterated. This was no longer a social call. "Did you eat breakfast yet?"

He looked at me hesitantly.

"Who ate that?" I asked, pointing to the tray.

He scratched his head and broke into a smile. "Guess I did."

His wife walked in with a Styrofoam cup of coffee from the hospital cafeteria and cheerily declared, "I'm back, dear." George looked at me with almost childlike innocence and said, "She's back." He did not recall her visit 15 minutes before. For a moment, I considered whether to examine George with his wife in the room. But it was best, I decided, to ease her into what I suspected by letting her overhear what was to come. Otherwise, she'd never believe the nature of this silent calamity.

I asked George to remember the words "peaches," "newspapers," and "Chestnut Street" and said that I'd ask him to repeat them in a few minutes. In the meantime I gave him a phone number and asked him to repeat it immediately, forward, and in reverse. This he did easily. He knew the name of the vice president and governor, recalled the places he and his wife had visited on a trip to Hawaii several weeks before the heart attack, slowly generated a list of ten words that began with the letter f, and copied a figure of a circle overlapping a rectangle. But when I asked him to recall the three words I had given him, he looked at me blankly.

I tried again with three words that are easy to associate— "school," "pencil," and "book." He repeated them 15 seconds later but had forgotten them within less than two minutes. Nor could he now remember the simple drawing he had just copied. George's language and perceptual skills were fine, and his memory for immediate and past events was intact. But he could not learn anything new. He suffered an anterograde amnesia. He drew from his past and registered the present, but his brain could not consolidate a new experience and retain it.

I walked his wife into the corridor and explained what I thought had happened. George had suffered a stroke in each of the temporal lobes, within the two coiled sea horse-shaped hippocampi. These swirls of nerve cells are especially susceptible to a critical fall in cerebral blood flow, and his plugged basilar artery made them even more vulnerable. They are the electrical switches that turn on our memory so we can record what we experience, and then somehow code this new information and send it off to the appropriate brain area to be stored for long-term memory. George had lost this pivotal step; he could not encode and retrieve anything that had just happened. I hoped he would improve.

To look for evidence of a stroke, I ordered a magnetic resonance scan. As soon as I recognized the bright crescents engraved into each of George's hippocampi on the scan, I felt the thrill of having made the correct diagnosis of a rare condition. But the horror of the problem, and maybe my guilt about okaying the surgery, quickly chilled any self-congratulation.

Pencil and paper tests given by a psychologist confirmed that, despite a normal IQ and intellect, a portion of George's memory was failing. His declarative memory—the type that we use to acquire and consciously recall facts and events—was letting him down. He would forget after 15 seconds what someone with a normal memory should be able to recall for a day. He held on to what had happened before the heart surgery and lived within the present, starting over perhaps every minute. It was as if the brain's tape recorder for life's experiences was set on an ebb and flow of automatic erase after every brief recording.

George and his wife have visited me monthly since the accident. At first, she thought he was sometimes faking the severity of his amnesia. Gradually, she stopped denying what was so difficult to believe. She took him to her office on days when he did not have therapy and sat him on a couch while she worked. We set up a cognitive rehabilitation program that tried to aid him with mnemonic strategies. Nothing helped much, but he did gain more insight into his memory failure.

On a recent late-afternoon visit, George wore his best square-dancing clothes, with polished boots and hair neatly slicked back. Surprised, I asked what he had been up to.

He shrugged and said, "Today? I got up and got here." He laughed.

"Anything else?" I pushed.

"You know. I get up, shower, eat breakfast, and go to the office or watch TV. We take our youngest son to school, I guess. Not sure when. I mean, I'm aware of today and so forth, but tomorrow I'll forget it."

His wife added, "He keeps asking for the time or date, again and again all day. He's even eaten breakfast two or three times in a morning, each time as if it's the first. And he follows me everywhere." She sounded irritated and frustrated, then suddenly perked up. "He keeps saying he wants to live in Hawaii. We went there before the stroke and twice after. He had a good time. Of course, he stayed right by me. Otherwise, he panics if I go where he can't see me. So he keeps telling me we should move there, but he doesn't recall our last two vacations in Hawaii."

"I like Hawaii," George interjected. "I don't have to see anyone I know there. I get a headache listening to people. They don't finish their sentences. I feel like I'm in a box, hearing little bits and pieces."

"Do you understand why this has happened?" I asked.

"I had a stroke. I get a headache when I think about it. Do you think I'll get my memory back?"

"You're getting better," I hedged, recalling the tubes, the ventilator, the failing heart, and the coma. "You remember some of what happens, especially if it carries emotional weight. Remember the earthquake?"

"Uh, San Francisco. I always used to go back there. Lived there when I was younger."

"You went through a lot in the hospital, and it takes time to get well," I said, as much for his wife, who could hang on to my words, as for my patient, who could not. George looked terribly sad. His wife took his hand. I realized how much more apathetic he had grown over the year. "When is my mind coming back?" he asked his wife. "I get a headache when I think about things."

George had a wisp of memory, like the remnants of a nightmare. But for the rest of us his personal nightmare would never fade away.

Bruce H. Dobkin, MD, FRCP, is Medical Director of the UCLA Neurologic Rehabilitation and Research Program.

CHAPTER

32

MECHANIC OF THE MIND

By Bruce Dobkin

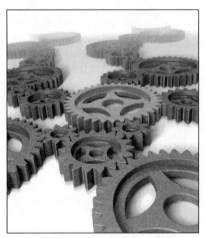

Photo 32-1

Harry straightened up after fiddling under the hood—the car's bonnet, he called it—and began, "It's those hoses. The um, um . . ." His eyes stole from mine to point above my brow, almost the way a schizophrenic focuses beyond the listener to see what is not really there. "Um, the rubber," he said. And then he started over with greater intensity. "The rubber deteriorates beneath the clamps and gas leaks out when she's cold."

Out of self-conscious vanity, I smoothed my hand across my forehead and, feeling nothing unusual, continued with a sweep of my fingers through my hair. Harry had done it again. He'd hesitate or stutter for a moment, trying to find a word on the tip of his tongue, and then—with a glance at my receding hairline—seemingly pick up a cue and continue his sentence. He had given me that same studied look several times before when I had brought my car to his repair shop, but I had pretended not to notice. I didn't want to put my neurologist's foot in my mouth, as I was often tempted to do when I noted a stranger with an odd limp or twitch that might signify a brain problem. Harry, after all, was probably getting medical advice elsewhere.

Still, I couldn't help but wonder whether he had an aphasia, a problem in the operation of the brain's language system. Every year 20 percent of the tens of thousands of people who suffer a stroke or a serious blow to the head will have to contend with a disturbance in a skill they always took for granted: their ability to speak fluently and comprehend what they hear and read. Language deficits can also occur as memory begins to fail in Alzheimer's disease. And frequent slips of the tongue may be the first warning sign of a tumor growing on the brain's left side, which houses our language centers.

But Harry, ever the polite British émigré, was onto me. "Sorry about that," he apologized. "Just vapor lock. Had to type it out." The crow's-feet about his eyes wrinkled deeper, and he smiled rather bashfully. "Bet you haven't tinkered with anything like this before," he said. I urged him on. I was hooked.

Twelve years ago, about three weeks after having coronary bypass surgery, Harry had suddenly become mute. He understood what others said and he could read with normal comprehension, but two days went by before he could speak at all. Even then he could not complete a sentence without stammering over at least one of the words he was trying to dredge up. To judge by his account, Harry had suffered a stroke on his brain's left side.

We walked away from the six hydraulic car lifts in his odorless, brightly lit garage with with its pristine white-tiled floors and made our way back to his office. His wife, a cheerful English woman in her sixties, answered phones and kept the books. She greeted me and asked about my twin daughters. After a few polite words, I turned back to Harry. He leaned towards me across his desk and began an extraordinary tale.

Two months after the bypass, he had returned to his auto-repair and yacht-rebuilding business, but his speech had gotten no better. It deteriorated to babble whenever he became upset or had the slightest argument or misunderstanding with an employee or customer. "He'd get so angry when he stumbled on a word," his wife broke in, "but I didn't know what was wrong. He kept it all to himself."

I wondered if Harry would have revealed what followed had I not been a doctor. His face turned almost crimson as he described his mounting frustration with his inability to say what was on his mind. One day, after another embarrassing dialogue with an old client, he found himself in tears, hiding in a corner of his shop. "I had lost all confidence," he said. "As a boy in boarding school, I was taught never to let others know your feelings." He threw up his hands. "But I couldn't communicate at all," he continued. "And I was too proud to make a fool of myself." He closed his business.

I understand why he had given up. Language is the faculty that, more than any other, makes us human. Indeed it is a relatively new skill. The ability to string together sounds and symbols for communication has existed for only a few tens of thousands of years. Many aphasics come to feel incompetent even though their overall intelligence, as measured by an intelligence quotient, does not decline. Those with insight into their impairment always anguish over their flubbed attempts to say what they mean. One of my patients, who could only say "yes, yes" a year after her stroke, once described her feelings to me by drawing a picture of herself as a mummy entombed in a bird cage.

Harry had never before seen himself as a failure. As if to convince me of the profound turnaround, he talked about his life before the stroke. As a young man, he had learned about engines from Sir Malcom Campbell, who let Harry work on his stable of world-class racing cars. He also became an accomplished musician. He built airplane engines during the war and later flew refugees into Palestine, raced autos in the 1950s, and then designed engines and boats before setting up his British auto shop in Los Angeles. There, customers chatted with Harry about cars and life while their automobiles were coddled in his white-tiled emporium. Until he quit.

Neurologists approach the complaints of their patients by trying to figure out which part of the brain their symptoms might arise from. Over a half-dozen kinds of aphasia were first pigeonholed by correlating the impairment people encounter after a brain injury with the damage later observed upon autopsy. A great deal more has since been learned through brain imaging techniques such as computerized tomography, positron emission tomography, and magnetic resonance, as well as by direct electric stimulation of the brain in patients being prepared for brain surgery. Harry had given me just enough information to picture the location of the hole that the stroke had punctured in his brain.

In cases of global aphasias, the most profound instances of language failure, the victim is unable to communicate or make sense of verbal and written language. Massive left-brain injuries to the frontal, temporal, and parietal lobes often lead to catastrophe. In Wernicke's aphasia, the unsuspecting patient yaks on, substituting meaningless or bizarre words for the correct ones. Even worse, he often has no insight into these errors and comprehends little of what others say. The lesion, in this case, is at the top of the temporal lobe, close to the parietal area. In Broca's aphasia, which results from injury to the frontal lobe and surrounding areas, the sufferer understands most of what others say, but his own output takes tremendous effect and produces only halting, disjointed phrases. Harry was mute for a day or two after his stroke, then had many of the deficiencies of a Broca's aphasia, suggesting that the damage had been done in the frontal areas of his brain.

Classic syndromes have added to our insights about brain and language. For example, some aphasics are word-deaf. They cannot point to a telephone when given the word, although they recognize the sound of a telephone and might name it after it rings—which suggests that there is more than one way to access the same word. Others are word-blind. They can write a spoken word, but cannot read the word they've just written. Still others might not be able to name, say, a cat upon seeing it, but after making appropriate associations—it purrs and is furry to touch—they manage to retrieve the animal's name by some alternate route.

I wondered whether Harry sometimes searched for a word by making similar associations in his mind. If so, the connections he made didn't always get him quite the right word. On one such occasion I recalled, he'd said "principate" when he meant to say "participate." So Harry had probably started out with a Broca's aphasia, then reached his present plateau of recovery with a barely noticeable problem in finding some of the words that might not come up in everyday conversation. What intrigued me was how he'd managed to improve so much after giving up on himself.

Actually, Harry told me, for four years he had tried to run away from the problem. He skied, flew gliders, and traveled around the world, avoiding all the most basic conversation with everyone, including his wife. Alone much of the time and unable to understand what was wrong, she left him. His deepening isolation led to a severe depression. Sequestered in a small hotel in Europe, he finally decided to find a way to help himself.

The way he tells it, he was lying in bed, staring at a pale wall, when he first attempted to visualize words before speaking them. If a word failed him, he pictured the object instead and then the printed word that symbolized it. In another exercise, he taught himself to mentally flash a card displaying the word he was about to use. Six weeks later he began to type out in his mind's eye the phrases that he was about to utter, and then he said them aloud as if he were reading from a teleprompter.

I imagine that his race driver's instincts helped here. Under pressure in a race, he'd been used to thinking ahead—simultaneously computing his position and speed relative to the other cars in the field so as to anticipate his next move. Years of reading blueprints had probably helped to hone his perceptual abilities as well.

He practiced mundane conversations on strangers, using their foreheads as his flashcards. "I could stay about eight bars ahead of what I was saying," the musician in him confided. "But I found that I had to keep the rhythm of speech going to keep from stalling out completely, until I could visualize the word. That's the 'um, um' you've probably noticed." Instinctively, it seemed, Harry had hit upon a compensatory mechanism that I had seen work in other patients. The right brain, which colors our speech with cadence and emotion, can apparently help certain aphasics produce proper phrases if they are trained to sing words rhythmically.

Then Harry upped the ante and resumed chatting with mechanics about technical matters. He practiced at this real-life drawing board until he had perfected his system. Within a few months he had reunited with his wife and reopened his auto shop. Over the past few years he'd become far more fluent and resorted to typing out words on foreheads only when emotionally upset or a lapse of connection or fatigue threw him off.

Harry and I walked back to my car with the new six-inch rubber hoses needed to replace the ones that had rotted. "So what do you think is going on in my brain circuits?" he asked.

As he told his story of recovery, I had imagined the cerebral center for language lighting up on the left side of his brain in the way they do with positron-emission tomography. With this technology, slightly radioactive substances injected into the blood allow us to see which parts of the brain become activated when we carry out a specific task. When we're presented with a written word, word-reading centers in the brain and around the occipital lobe at the back of the brain light up as they increase their blood flow and activity. When we're asked to define a word, a portion of the left frontal lobe becomes active. When we hear words spoken, the temporal lobe's so-called auditory cortex lights up, along with a nearby patch of the left parietal lobe. Each of these areas is made up of tens of millions of neurons and connected by pathways over which nerve messages travel at lightning speed to coordinate the complex activities of language. Until recently, neuroscientists had no good evidence that the adult brain could remodel these connections after injury, or at least shift some of the work done by a damaged site to a still-functioning community of neurons. But studies now suggest that the brain can reorganize its pathways, so it may be possible to find treatment that promotes recovery.

Most aphasics improve measurably for a year or more following their left-brain injury. After his stroke, much of Harry's improvement came from his self-taught strategy of visualizing words and drawing on associations. Perhaps he worked around the path that was disconnected, making use of another route to the "lost and found" of words, or stimulated his brain to build another pathway.

As Harry replaced the eroded rubber connectors that leaked gasoline on my car's engine, he mentioned something about the heart surgery and stumbled, mumbling "um, um, um" before finding the elusive word on my forehead. "Did it again," he said. "Did you catch it?" I nodded, but I might have applauded. Harry had intuitively tinkered with the connections for language under his bonnet and had come up with a way to pull cerebral pathways together as cleverly as he would restore the links in my failing car.

Bruce H. Dobkin, MD, FRCP, is Medical Director of the UCLA Neurologic Rehabilitation and Research Program.

CHAPTER

33

THE ABSENTMINDED PROFESSOR

By Bruce H. Dobkin

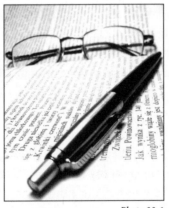

Photo 33-1

The professor of anthropology from a nearby college could barely contain his irritation. He quickly made it clear that this neurological consultation was for the benefit of his wife alone. She had nagged him for years about what she called his "unfitting behavior." After the car accident, his physician suggested they see me to settle the matter.

This was not an auspicious start.

The professor fully looked the part of an old-school academician in a brown corduroy sport coat with suede elbow patches, wrinkled khaki pants, scuffed Vibram-soled shoes, and thinning white hair brushed back from his temples. In measured phrases tinged with a remnant of a North Carolina accent—held on to despite forty years of teaching in southern California—he described the accident.

"I was backing out into the street from a parking lot," he began. "I might have heard a rasping sound, and my wife was saying something, but for whatever reason, I wasn't paying close attention. So I stopped the car and she drove. I did apparently scrape the passenger side."

His wife pursed her lips and folded her hands on the lap of a pleated tartan skirt. Looking at her white blouse with its Peter Pan collar, I imagined that her wardrobe had changed little from her days as a college student in the 1940s. She seemed to require my permission to speak. I nodded.

"Well, Robert, there was more to it than that," she opened cautiously. "You drove in reverse down a line of three parked cars and ignored my calls to stop. Then you put the car in forward and drove for two more blocks—and through a stop sign. I was frantic and begged you to stop, but you completely ignored me. After I asked you for the tenth time to pull over, you finally looked at me and turned into the gardening store's parking lot. When I showed you the damage to our car and said that we had to go back and leave a note for the people whose cars you'd hit, all you could say was, 'Whatever pleases you.'"

The professor sat beside my desk and stared steadily at an ophthalmoscope on the wall above an exam table. "Do you recall this?" I asked.

He said nothing. I was about to repeat the question when he squinted his eyes, as if weighing whether what she said made any sense. "Well, she may be exaggerating my seeming lack of interest," he said.

"Did you feel anything unusual at the time, perhaps a bit bewildered?" I asked.

After a few more long moments he replied, "Well, I might have felt a little lost in space."

I began to probe into his past. Before the accident, had he ever seemed unaware of what he was doing? He said no, but his wife quickly brought up the faculty dinner 17 years earlier at which they'd announced their engagement. At the dinner table, she recounted, he had turned to her and mumbled something, then slowly leaned forward until his face fell into the fettuccine on his plate. No one said anything. She and his department chairman pulled him up by the shoulders; he seemed befuddled for a moment, then told them he felt fine.

"What did you make of this?" I asked the professor.

"She told me about it while wiping some sauce off my face, and I figured that I'd had too much to drink." He shrugged his shoulders.

At the most, he drank two glasses of wine, his wife countered. But no one at the table seemed surprised. And when I took him to see a doctor the next day, his cardiogram and blood tests were normal. The doctor told us that he'd probably passed out from the alcohol.

Next I asked if he'd had any other spells like this, or other car accidents. Again he said no. Again his wife disagreed. "What about the time you slammed your foot on the brakes at a cross street, even though you had the right of way, and we were rear-ended?" she reminded him with some bitterness. "I had pain from the whiplash for months."

"I mean that I don't think I've ever passed out like that before," he replied.

"No, not exactly," she agreed. "But I'll tell you something, and you either pay no attention or bring up an entirely unrelated subject, as if I didn't exist. And you do terribly impolite things, and instead of apologizing you insist—not without anger—that I'm misunderstanding or overstating the case."

He had obviously heard this before. "I've told you that I get absorbed and mean no disrespect," he said. "Even the marriage counselor has said we both have to be more patient with each other's little habits."

So, I thought, there's more to this than medicine. Domestic squabbling was obviously playing a role here, and this couple wanted me to help their counselor restore goodwill. The real problem might be nothing other than a wife who expects more in the way of decent manners from a scholar who is dedicated to studying the manners of other cultures.

At the same time, the professor's wife was trying hard not to be personally insulted by his behavior. She mentioned that his previous wife had divorced him shortly after their last child left for college in upstate New York—a bit of information meant to let me know that he had never been easy to live with. Still, no matter how moody, meditative, or aloof he might be or always had been, I needed to settle for myself whether or not a neurological problem existed. And to do that I needed to ask more questions.

I started with the wife. "Can you give me some examples of what he does that you find out of the ordinary?"

Without a pause she said, "He'll repeatedly tap his spoon against the bottom of his soup bowl. I mean, for two or three minutes before even taking a sip, and then he might do it again."

"It's only for a second or two," he interrupted.

"No, it's for minutes, and when I ask you to stop you ignore me. And when you've finally stopped and seem more inclined to listen to what I'm saying, you lash out at me."

I then asked him whether he was aware of brief spells when he might lose track of a conversation or falter as he lectured. Did he often experience a peculiar sense of déjà vu or of feeling disconnected from his world? After each question he paused in thought, then gave me a definitive no.

I turned back to his wife. "Does he ever stare off into space and repetitively blink his eyes, smack his lips, or do some other stereotyped movement—something like the spoon tapping?"

"No, I don't think so. But he'll walk in front of me or step on the heel of my shoe and trip me and seem oblivious to what he's done." Her husband looked steadily ahead, offering no defense. "And there was the time I was standing on some phone books on top of a wobbly chair trying to dust out a cobweb up on the ceiling. He was holding the chair and had me by the waist. Suddenly, without a word, he let go and walked away and I lost my balance and fell. My leg was killing me. I screamed to him to call 911. He continued to walk toward the bathroom. When I yelled again, he came out and I begged him to call an ambulance. He lifted the phone and, without dialing, said something like, 'They can't come.' Then he stood over me for maybe a minute before he knelt down to help. Finally he went and made the call. My hip was broken and I spent a week in the hospital. It still bothers me, eight years later."

"What do you make of this?" I asked him.

"I recall the situation, but I'm not clear on some of the details," he answered. "I mean, I must have had to go to the bathroom and then didn't think fast enough to realize she was hurt."

His wife wasn't ready to let him explain it away that easily. "But he does do these odd things, and it gets him angry if I make a fuss," she protested. "I let most of the incidents go by so he won't get upset." I waited for her to go on, but she was suddenly busily attending to a loose skirt thread.

It was obvious that she wanted to state her case, but without accusing her prominent husband of being mean, inconsiderate, or even bizarre. And though she seemed to sense this might help me explain his lapses in civil behavior—which she estimated to occur about once a week— she seemed reluctant to provide me with greater detail. Maybe she didn't want to add anything that could further threaten their marriage. Maybe her husband had at times acted in a way so offensive she dared not confront him or leak the information to a doctor.

With this suspicion in mind, I encouraged her to push past her strong sense of propriety. "When he seems to ignore you, has he ever acted in a way that might embarrass either of you?"

She paused, finally touching her hand to his and saying, "Robert, don't take this personally," before she turned to me. "Yes. On many occasions over the years, he'll start to . . . well . . . he'll pick his nose. I mean, he'll take one finger after the other, the ring and pinkie on his left hand, and put one in his nose, lick it, then put the other in and lick that and continue this, sometimes for several minutes. If I ask him what he's doing, he either won't answer or says, 'I don't know.'"

"I don't really do that, do I?" He looked puzzled.

"You do," she answered firmly, "and one of the times was when we were at the president's faculty reception surrounded by friends. No one pays attention, because they all consider you to be so eccentric anyway."

It was this final detail that gave me my diagnosis. The nose-picking behavior was so antisocial, so out of character, and seemingly beyond his control, that it fell beyond eccentricity. In ancient times, the professor would have been deemed possessed. Today, he would be called an epileptic.

While most people picture an epileptic seizure as so violent and extreme that it can hardly go unnoticed, I explained to the professor and his wife that he might well be having these attacks of altered awareness due to a type of seizure called partial complex, or psychomotor. A virtual storm of electrical discharges was coming from the neurons of one of the brain's temporal lobes, where new memories are formed and many of the pathways for emotions reside. In a partial complex seizure, for reasons no one really understands, this outbreak of abnormal brain activity could result in the professor's unwilled behaviors as well as his amnesia concerning these simple acts. Normally, each neuron's firing rate is influenced and modified by its neighboring cells, but in the professor's case, an old head injury, tumor, or stroke could have isolated a particular patch of nerve cells from their neighbors, allowing the patch to occasionally fire without restraint. For the seconds or minutes when such a storm clouded over his awareness, the professor became an automaton who could trip his wife or leave her writhing on the floor, sideswipe three cars without knowing it, or tap, pick, and stare in a maddening fashion. Then, as the seizure ceased, his mind drifting in a confused, amnesiac state, he would lash out at his wife.

Remarkably, the professor readily accepted my tentative diagnosis. He liked its logic, even if he couldn't offer, or remember, any evidence in its favor. His wife seemed relieved and asked me to talk to their counselor.

I ordered an electroencephalogram for the professor, to monitor his brain's electrical waves. I hoped it might show us some epileptic activity, though he would have to have a seizure during the EEG in order for it to be detected. A magnetic resonance scan would show us if he had any serious brain disorder.

I quickly assured him, however, that the cause was not likely to be a malignant tumor, since I suspected he'd been having these lapses of consciousness even before he married his present wife. I asked him to discuss the matter with his children and former wife. Was it possible he'd been having these spells for decades?

In the meantime, however, the most practical way to determine whether or not the professor had epilepsy would be to put him on anticonvulsant medication. If he stopped having attacks while on the drug, then my diagnosis would be secure. In addition, I told him not to drive a car until we were certain the seizures had stopped. I would have bet that the only reason he'd never had a really serious accident was that he had walked to work for 30 years and rarely drove on the freeways. Indeed, if the diagnosis proved correct, we could all be thankful that no greater harm had come to the couple while he was under the influence of the electrical demon.

The professor and his wife returned several weeks later. His tests had all come back normal, which was not surprising since he didn't have a seizure during the EEG. In some instances, a patient can be continuously monitored by an EEG and simultaneously videotaped in an attempt to tie his behavior to a spell. For the professor, that didn't seem necessary.

Bruce H. Dobkin, MD, FRCP, is Medical Director of the UCLA Neurologic Rehabilitation and Research Program.

CHAPTER

34

FIGHTING WITH PHANTOMS

By Bruce H. Dobkin

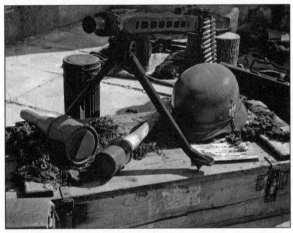

Photo 34-1

George zeroed in on my eyes when I looked up from his neatly typed page of notes. In three paragraphs he had matter-of-factly described the skirmish that had taken place in the plane's lavatory. "We'll immediately pursue all the tests you order," he said briskly. His wife nodded her assent, with a look of relief on her face.

"Your notes are very useful," I assured him. "But I'd like to get more of the flavor of how the episode unfolded. It might help us to decide how to proceed."

He pulled his shoulders back and assumed even more of a military brace. I asked if he had been in the service. A Hollywood casting director would have pegged him as a Marine colonel in his late 50s. "Oh," George said, "I was a bomber pilot in World War II, then a test pilot before becoming an engineer." At 70, he still ran his own consulting business as a troubleshooter for firms that sent him to military bases in other countries to solve technical problems with their aircraft.

He summarized his experience as precisely as he had written about it. On a commercial flight several days ago, he had closed the door to a restroom cubicle and tried to pull down his pants zipper. His right hand could not seem to find it. While struggling to unzip himself, he thought he heard someone trying to open the door behind him. Maybe it was just a little air turbulence, he conjectured. Suddenly he felt what seemed to be a hand pressing against the small of his back. Perhaps, he reasoned, it was just a chill from one of those tiny air jets by the sink.

But then he sensed that whatever had rattled the door was actually inside the cubicle. It slid like a snake around the right side of his waist. With his left hand he grabbed at something fleshy and hard and struggled for a few seconds to pull off the sinuous thing. It tightened its grasp around him, but he stood his ground over the toilet. Finally he yanked it up to eye level and saw what he had been wrestling with. He had been grappling with himself. His left hand was holding his own right forearm.

"I finished the zipper routine and went back to my seat without a problem," he said.

He mentioned nothing to his wife about the battle in the toilet and resumed work on an expense account. However, he repeatedly jotted the numbers down an inch or so outside the column in which he wanted them. No matter how hard he concentrated or how rigidly he propped his right wrist against his notepad, he could not squarely hit the two-inch column. "Figured it was just the shadows from the overhead lighting," he told me. He checked the angle of the light by blocking its beam with his right hand and realized that wherever he held it, he was missing the outer fingers. When he held his hand palm up, his right thumb disappeared. When he laid his hand palm down on the paper, the right thumb reappeared and the little and ring fingers vanished. About 15 minutes later, all the fingers gradually returned and he was able to place his accounting figures where he wanted them.

How did he feel about this bizarre event? "I wasn't frightened or especially concerned, but something wasn't right," he replied. The incident reminded him of his experiences while training to be a high-altitude pilot. "They'd put us into a decompression chamber and tell us to write until our skills deteriorated to the point where we could only scribble. I figured the plane lost pressurization while I was in the john and that had made my mind play tricks on me."

As a pilot, he would have known that in an unpressurized aircraft climbing faster than 1,000 feet per minute (or in equivalent conditions in a decompression chamber), people can start to falter when doing simple arithmetic at an altitude of only 10,000 feet. By 18,000 feet most people respond slowly, writing becomes illegible, and intellectual functions start to grow almost delusional, until at 20,000 to 25,000 feet, consciousness dissipates altogether.

However, George's rationalization fell short. Had his symptoms really been caused by sudden decompression in the plane's cabin, others—perhaps his wife—would also have experienced them. It was not until he and his wife landed and waited in a terminal for the flight that would take them home that he even mentioned the incident to her. I asked her how he had behaved.

"Nothing out of the ordinary," she remarked. She hadn't noticed any difficulty with his speech or thinking on the plane. And his balance and strength seemed normal when he got up from his seat and maneuvered their carry-on luggage off the aircraft. "He seemed a bit amused by it all when he finally told me," she said.

But she was clearly shocked by his admission. Not only was she now a psychologist, but she had previously been a nurse, so she could imagine all kinds of possible afflictions of the brain and mind, from dementia to psychosis to vascular disease, that might account for the events. She insisted that they see his physician the next day. The family internist, perplexed by his patient's symptoms, ordered a magnetic resonance imaging study of his brain. The images revealed a white crescent of swollen tissue extending below the surface of the grayish left cerebral hemisphere, at the junction of the sensory and visual cortex. George had suffered a stroke.

His peculiar symptoms were easier to make sense of given this narrow wedge of cortical injury. Transiently, perhaps for only minutes, that portion of the brain had been robbed of blood, oxygen, and nutrients. The nerve cells in this area participate in appreciating what the right side of the body feels and where the right arm and leg are in space. When they faltered, George's right chest and arm had been disconnected from his awareness of them. He thought he was using his right hand to unzip his pants, but actually it had assumed a life of its own beyond his conscious control and perception.

As blood drained away from these cortical areas, sensation ebbed like a shadow moving across his body's right side, leaving behind a cool, crawling feeling. His right field of vision had also disappeared in its wake. He saw only what one might view through goggles with the right half of each lens obscured by tape. So his right arm, the expense account column, and his fingers came into sight only when they rested in the left half of his world.

That was apparently why George could not at first recognize that the invisible alien around his waist was his own arm. It wasn't until he yanked the arm up to his left field of vision that he saw that it belonged to him. Although sensation soon returned to the right side of his body—he was able to zip up, leave the cubicle, and return to his seat as if nothing had happened—his vision took longer to recover. Another 15 minutes or so elapsed before he could plant his expense account numbers squarely in their column. Luckily, blood flow restored itself to prevent permanent destruction of his faculties.

George had several risk factors for vascular disease. His mother had died from a heart attack at age 58, and he'd inherited her high blood cholesterol. This led to his own atherosclerosis (a building up of fatty plaque inside his blood vessel walls), resulting in two silent heart attacks within the past 12 years. He had never had chest pain, or at least he'd never paid attention to any discomfort at the time of the attacks. Some routine tests by his physician picked up the damage to his heart wall after each event.

The tests paved the way to two coronary bypass surgeries. After the second one, almost a year ago, an infection in his chest wall required a surgeon to reopen his chest, sawing through the bony sternum, so the wound could be treated and heal. On his back in a hospital bed for a week, with his heart exposed under sterile dressings soaked in antibiotics, George watched the pulsation of his muscular pump.

Perhaps the atherosclerosis that had plugged his heart's arteries was now building up in one or more of the vessels to his brain, hampering blood flow there as well. Or perhaps prior damage to the heart wall might have allowed jellied clots of blood to form on it, break free, and travel up to the cerebral arteries until they proved too fat to pass any farther.

I wondered whether his nonchalant attitude about his alien arm and disappearing fingers came from an indifference stemming from his stroke; maybe a brain region that contributes to insight and emotional responsiveness had also been involved. In patients with right cerebral strokes, apathy and denial that anything is wrong is quite common—even if the left side of the body is paralyzed. Some even imagine that the insensate arm was stolen or floated out the window.

But such strange perceptual twists are rare with a left brain injury like the one George had. Then again, he was obviously a disciplined, stoic fellow. As a pilot during World War II, he had held his course under fire until the moment his payload of bombs had to be dropped. As a test pilot he had often faced uncertainty and managed to suppress surges of adrenalized fear. As a patient, he had calmly eyeballed his heart pumping in his chest without getting upset. Alarm over a novel experience was just not in his psychic wiring.

We proceeded to the studies that might tell us why he had this stroke and how we could prevent another, more serious one. We found no obvious answers. An ultrasound test that bounces sound waves off the chamber walls and valves of the heart revealed no clots or debris. And an initial scan of his carotid arteries, which run up the neck and into the brain, showed no definite narrowing of the blood vessels. He agreed to an arteriogram, an invasive and somewhat more precarious test that allows us to see blood circulating through the brain. The test in itself carries a small risk of causing a stroke.

In the darkened arteriography suite late the next day, I wore an apron with a lead core that barricaded me from the X-rays aimed at George during his test. He calmly chatted with us and held still under his green sterile drapes. The radiologist poked a plastic catheter into a blood vessel in George's groin and inched the wiry tube up the wide aorta in the belly and chest to the site where the carotids branch off and head for the brain. The 1 percent risk of a stroke comes from the chance that the catheter will nick an artery wall and flick off debris into the brain's circulation.

Once the catheter was in place, the radiologist injected dye into the bloodstream to help visualize the brain's vascular network. We could instantly see the images of each vessel and its serpiginous branches light up on a TV monitor. X-ray pictures, developed minutes later, revealed that several of his arteries contained irregular mounds of atherosclerosis that jutted into the bloodstream. We concluded that one of these plaques at the top of the left carotid, which extends two major branches into the brain, had probably caused his stroke. Most likely a piece of porridge-like material had spontaneously split off and briefly plugged a smaller, distant branch feeding into his cortical areas.

But now, three days after the event, we could no longer see any sign of the debris. Presumably, it had quickly disintegrated, restoring flow to the injured but not-yet-destroyed patch of cortex.

As the radiologist pulled out the catheter, I told George that the odds seemed against another imminent attack. But he'd always be at greater risk than another man his age who had been free of vascular disease. The only course was to continue keeping his risk factors under control. (Surgery to clean the artery wall was not an option: The most irregular plaques had accumulated beyond the easy-to-reach carotids in his neck.)

"You think I ought to retire and take it easy?" George asked, still on his back. "I do get myself into some stressful situations," he admitted, "though the wife and I make each trip out of the country into a working vacation."

I left it to him and his wife to decide. For a man like George, inactivity might seem like more stress than working.

George sat around the house for a few days, then left with his wife to see a customer in Asia. He would not retire. He'd live with the uncertainty that even his best effort might not prevent a serious stroke or heart attack. Coming to grips with that notion was no more trying than the wrestling match in the lavatory.

Bruce H. Dobkin, MD, FRCP, is Medical Director of the UCLA Neurologic Rehabilitation and Research Program.

35

NETTING THE BUTTERFLY

By Bruce H. Dobkin

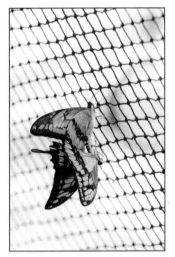

Photo 35-1

Thomas Wright sat stiffly and squinted at a blank wall in my examining room, as if trying to visualize the scenes his wife was reconstructing for me. The incidents were fixed firmly in her memory, but for him, they might not have existed at all.

It had all begun eight months earlier. Thinking back to that day, Mrs. Wright wondered if perhaps her husband had overdone his exercise: In the two years since retiring from his position as an executive with a supermarket chain, he had ridden a mountain bike for at least an hour every day. Could it have been fatigue that caused him to fall backward off a step stool while changing a light bulb in the garage? When she found him, he was unconscious, his head bathed in a pool of blood. She had pulled out a dish towel that was tucked into her apron, pressed it against his oozing scalp, and called the paramedics.

Doctors in the emergency room had sutured off the visible bleeders, but the real problem lay inside the skull. The jolt against the concrete floor had fractured that bony vault, leaving it cracked like the shell of a hard-boiled egg, with irregular lines and depressed islands. The trauma had torn blood vessels both on the surface and deep within his brain, bruising, shearing, and twisting his cerebral landscape with all the fury of a tornado. A CT scan revealed thin crescents of clotted blood between the skull and the surface of his brain's frontal lobes, as well as a clot over his left temporal lobe. Blotches of blood filled two dime-sized contusions deeper in his brain. As these bruises swelled, they pressed so dangerously against the area of the brain that controls breathing that his doctors decided to connect him to a mechanical ventilator.

He'd awakened the next day. "I called his name, and he opened his eyes and squeezed my hand," Mrs. Wright recalled. "I was so hopeful, in spite of the cautious prognosis given by the doctors. You see, Tom had an accident when he was a teenager. A car sideswiped his bicycle. The head injury that time affected his speech for some months, but it didn't keep him out of the war or out of college." Her tone of voice and earnest expression made it clear that she wanted me to know her husband had been an accomplished person, someone who was still worth trying to help.

I asked my new patient if he remembered anything about the accident, the hospital stay, or the six weeks of rehabilitation therapy. He turned to me with a smile that puckered the crow's-feet around his eyes. "Sometimes you don't remember all the things," he confided.

Next I asked him about the long scar running over the left side of his bald scalp. "Must have bumped the thing," he said. He began picking at a callus below his wedding band.

His wife's eyes reddened with tears. "Please," she said, defending his lapse. "I know his memory and the way he stumbles using words isn't good. I don't expect that will come back any more than it has. But he was doing better a month ago. Why?"

"Well, first tell me about how he has changed," I replied.

"It's little things, you know. He used to dress himself when I put out his clothes; he'd ask, 'What's for dinner?' when he was hungry—although, I'll admit, sometimes it was lunchtime—and we'd walk half a mile in the park every morning. Now he hardly does anything." She fiddled with the buttons on her red cardigan. It had an arrangement of purple, white, and yellow flowers on each side, with stitching loose enough to suggest that she had knit it herself. She looked up at me to deliver her real message. "If things get much worse, I won't be able to manage him at home."

"I understand," I assured her. I began searching for clues, for some insight into her husband's deterioration. "Do you think his walking has changed?" I asked. "Do his feet ever seem to get stuck?"

"No," she answered, curious about what I might be getting at. "I mean, he just doesn't seem to want to get around as much."

"Has he had any trouble holding his urine or bowels?"

"He goes to the bathroom when he has to. I don't believe he's ever wet himself."

With his barrel chest and muscular arms and calves, Thomas Wright looked more ready for a singles match on a tennis court than for a bed in a nursing home. As I began to examine him, however, I noticed that he was walking cautiously and ever so slightly scuffing the toes of his right foot on the ground as he swung that leg forward. When I tested the individual muscles, I found a trace of weakness in his right arm and leg, a residue of the trauma to the left side of his brain; because of that weakness, he had a mild limp.

His cognitive troubles, on the other hand, were not at all mild. He could not name the month and guessed that the year was 1978. When I told him the date, he forgot it a minute or two later. He could spell "cat" forward but not in reverse. He immediately repeated the names of three items that I asked him to remember but could not recall any of them, even with some clues, a minute later. He did not know his own date of birth or the names of his three children. "Who can keep up?" he mused. I asked him to give me a list of ten animals, but all he could come up with was "zoo whatchamacallits." He could tell me the names of only about half the common objects and parts of the body that I pointed to. The word "thigh," for instance, eluded him. Mrs. Wright sighed sadly when instead of copying the box I had drawn he penciled only three oddly intersected lines. When I asked him to connect, in alphabetical order, scattered circles containing letters from A to L, he knew to draw a line between A and B but appeared stumped by the next move.

In all, the examination took less than an hour, but it was all the time I needed to map the landscape of Mrs. Wright's anguish. The cerebral tornado had left in its wake a man with the equivalent of a severe case of Alzheimer's disease.

There should have been one major difference, however. The intellectual decline of people with Alzheimer's gets inexorably steeper. Mr. Wright's deterioration should have halted shortly after the accident.

I reviewed the three-inch pile of evaluations from speech and physical therapists and the reports made by his physicians. The only difference between what had been written three months earlier and what I had just seen was that back then he had been described as frustrated by his errors. Now he seemed resigned or unconcerned. I began to wonder whether the changes his wife had chronicled might simply reflect a darkening of his mood. Could Mr. Wright have become so depressed by his constant failures that he was withdrawing from a life he no longer understood?

Next I looked at the half-dozen radiology studies of his brain taken during the first days after the accident and then two and six months later. They showed that the clots had gradually disappeared, but patchy wedges of destroyed gray and white matter persisted. That was bad news: These tissue injuries made it impossible for Mr. Wright to take full advantage of his brain's resources for language, memory, attention span, and judgment.

The scans did, however, raise the possibility of a sometimes treatable diagnosis. I noticed that his cerebral ventricles, the dark, butterfly-shaped, fluid-filled caverns in the center of the brain, had enlarged modestly over time. The ventricles produce about 30 tablespoonfuls of clear spinal fluid a day; slow currents move the fluid through a narrow channel out to the surface, where it bathes and cushions the brain and spinal cord. Normally, about the same amount of fluid that's created is absorbed by the surface of the brain. If it's not removed as fast as it's produced, the pool grows and the ventricles begin to enlarge, pushing aside the rather elastic tissue of the surrounding brain. The nerve fibers compressed by the expanding pool are those that play a role in walking, memory, and bladder control. The disease—the excess spinal fluid and the trouble that fluid causes—is called hydrocephalus, literally meaning water in the head.

Most often, when we think of hydrocephalus, we think of babies with large heads. Their hydrocephalus generally occurs when the outlet channels that direct the fluid from the ventricles to the brain's surface fail to develop. But hydrocephalus can also be the result of tumors that compress or obstruct the fluid's flow. Sometimes a head injury or bleeding damages the delicate, spongy tissues that cover the surface of the brain so that they cannot absorb the fluid. In any of these cases, the ventricles begin to expand and symptoms begin to appear—symptoms that could explain the kind of deterioration Thomas Wright was experiencing.

After I had told Mr. and Mrs. Wright about the condition, I explained that there is only one way to get the fluid that is produced and that which needs to be removed back into equilibrium. A neurosurgeon drills a tiny hole through the skull and passes a thin plastic tube into one of the butterfly wings. A one-way valve directs the excess fluid to the other end of this shunt, which is placed in the patient's belly. The now-decompressed butterfly gradually shrinks back to its normal size.

"Would he get a little better or, I mean, could he get back to being himself?" Mrs. Wright asked.

I told her that if her husband indeed had hydrocephalus, the shunt should enable him to regain the ground he had lost in the last few months. But, I added, there was no test I could do to predict with certainty how he would respond. All too often after a serious head injury like his, the ventricles are enlarged only because the rest of the brain has withered around them. And that's not hydrocephalus: the butterfly is simply spreading its wings to fill the vacuum. In such a case, merely shunting fluid away would have little effect on the permanent brain damage wrought by the injury.

So, I explained, before recommending the surgery doctors want to be as sure as they can that the patient is indeed suffering from hydrocephalus. And what gives them the most certainty in that diagnosis is seeing a particular triad of symptoms: memory loss, incontinence, and a peculiar problem with walking called an apraxia, in which the person's feet seem to stick to the ground as he tries to take a step. Mr. Wright's case wasn't nearly so clear. His ventricles were not as large as I had seen in other patients who responded to a shunt, his memory loss could well be due solely to the brain trauma he'd sustained at the time of his fall, his walking was not typical of apraxia, and he was not incontinent. "In other words," I told the couple, "pursuing a shunt would mean betting on a long shot that carried a 10 percent risk of a potentially life-threatening complication—like the introduction of bacteria that cause meningitis, a disease in which the membranes surrounding the brain and spinal cord become inflamed."

Having given them all the hard facts I could, I told them it might be best simply to hold off on a decision for a while, to see if the typical triad of symptoms evolved. Mrs. Wright immediately agreed: She said she wasn't ready to try something that might

NETTING THE BUTTERFLY 235

hurt him. Before they left, I gave Mr. Wright a prescription for an antidepressant, to lift his mood and be sure that it wasn't affecting his concentration, memory, and drive.

Three weeks later, I got a call from Mrs. Wright. She said that her husband was much worse. He could hardly walk and he was wetting himself. Although these new symptoms did indeed complete the triad, I wanted to make sure that they were not the result of the antidepressant medication. Even the low dose Mr. Wright was taking could spark these sorts of side effects in his traumatized brain. So I asked Mrs. Wright to stop giving him the pills and to watch for the symptoms to begin clearing. When she pushed him and his new wheelchair into my office a week later, I knew discontinuing the medicine hadn't done the trick.

"I can't keep him at home this way," she said. "He's like a baby and getting worse every day."

As for Mr. Wright, he seemed to have no idea what was happening. "What can I help you with?" I asked him.

"Oh, just visiting," he answered.

"What kind of work do I do?" I tugged at the lapels of my white coat.

"Good question," he smiled.

I helped him stand up and told him to walk through the doorway. His body leaned forward slightly, but his feet stayed glued to the ground. I gave him a gentle nudge while holding on to his belt at the small of his back; he took two steps like an ox whose feet were stuck in deep mud. Then he stopped, and urine ran down onto his shoes. He had the triad, all right. But did he have the disease?

"What about that operation?" Mrs. Wright asked sadly. It was her only hope, she explained, and I agreed. If she were to place him in a nursing home, this helpless man would most likely die from bedsores and infections.

I admitted him to the hospital and ordered yet another set of MRI images. When I looked at them and compared them with the older studies, the butterfly's wings were at best only slightly larger. So I called one of my neurosurgical colleagues and described Mr. Wright's case. "Sounds like there's nothing much left to lose," he said.

The surgery went smoothly. Three days later Mr. Wright took a few steps with less of the inertia that had held him back in my office the week before. He was still quite unsteady, however, and just as confused. To buy his wife some time before she had to become a full-time caretaker again, I arranged for ten days of inpatient rehabilitation therapy.

A week after Thomas Wright's release from the hospital, he opened the door of my exam room, motioned his wife to walk in, and strode in behind her. According to the smiling Mrs. Wright, he now dressed and fed himself, walked four blocks a day with her, and was logging half an hour each day on his stationary bicycle. When I examined him I found that, remarkably, his right-side weakness had improved and his walking was only slightly wobbly. Even more amazing, he could more easily retrieve information stored in his memory. He recalled the words "red," "cabbage," and "Oldsmobile" a few minutes after I said them, although I did have to remind him that one was a color, one a vegetable, and one a car.

There was one intriguing change—Mr. Wright had developed some odd rituals. For example, Mrs. Wright told me how, that morning, he had torn all the sheets off a roll of toilet paper and neatly stacked them on the sink. I asked him about the toilet paper business.

"Oh, I get onto it and it goes," he replied, perhaps not so cryptically. It seemed that once something captured his attention, his still-damaged frontal lobes—responsible for a number of behaviors, including sifting out what's important from what isn't—wouldn't let him see past it.

But although many words and memories still eluded him, the shunt had restored more of his cognition than I would have predicted. In retrospect, I realized that the hydrocephalus must have been working insidiously against him from the beginning, as he tried to recover from the acute effects of the brain trauma.

"What's that bump along your head?" I asked, as my finger traced the subcutaneous route of the shunt and its soft valve.

"Oh, operated on to a degree, I suppose," he answered.

Bruce H. Dobkin, MD, FRCP, is Medical Director of the UCLA Neurologic Rehabilitation and Research Program.

CHAPTER

36

AN INSULT TO THE BRAIN

By Bruce H. Dobkin

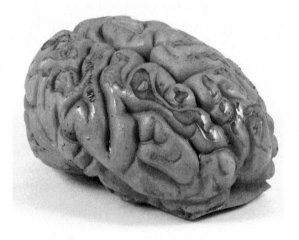

Photo 36-1

The receptionist's note about my next patient read, "Rear-ended two months ago—whiplash. Headaches, irritable, not herself. Referred by boss."

Terrific, I thought. A straightforward whiplash injury, not another university medical center second-opinion case with a four-inch stack of records. The impact of the collision had probably stretched and twisted the woman's neck muscles as well as ligaments and joints along the spine. Proper physical therapy mixed, if needed, with a bit of medication would melt away the tender and sprained areas and the headache pain they transmit. Then I made out the less legible words that followed: "No mental agility." Maybe I had jumped the gun.

Nancy turned her head and shoulders at the same time, like a statue rotating on a lazy Susan, as she explained what had happened. She had pulled onto the freeway at rush hour and stayed in the outside lane, where a heavy line of traffic was moving at about 30 miles an hour. A few minutes later, the car in front of her braked to a stop. As Nancy slowed to a halt, she glanced in her rearview mirror and saw a pickup truck bearing down on her. She clutched the steering wheel and the truck slammed into her, throwing her body forward and back. She remembered crying out "Oh, no!" as she careened into the car ahead. After that jolt, she was hit again from behind and again lurched forward against her seat belt and back.

Moments later, someone knocked on her windshield and asked if she was okay. Nancy looked into her rearview mirror, which now tilted toward her awkwardly. The nose and mouth it reflected seemed unfamiliar. Her foot brushed against a coffee mug holder with a sandbag bottom. It must have fallen off the console, she thought. She gradually connected the holder with the collision, then heard someone ask again, "Are you okay?"

She rolled down her window. "I will be," she answered. But she wanted to sleep.

Nancy pulled over and waited, unsure about what should happen next. After a while a highway patrol officer came by, asked how she felt, and asked to see her license and registration. She thought about what he had said. He explained, for the second time, that he needed her license and registration for his report; then he asked which lane she had been in. A picture drawn by her six-year-old niece came to mind: a red bus on a single lane surrounded by green hills. "If the fast lane is number one, which one were you in?" he asked softly. She looked at him as if he had posed an impossibly difficult mathematical problem. He repeated the question. She studied the traffic that dribbled past, deliberately counted the lanes, and answered four. Because she had been so slow to respond, the officer called an ambulance.

When the paramedics finally arrived, they checked her blood pressure, asked her the date and the name of the governor, and flashed a light into her eyes. No apparent injuries, they said, but her muscles might feel real stiff tomorrow. Nancy thanked them, then took a look around her car. The headlights were cracked and the trunk was sprung open. She tied the trunk shut with a wire clothes hanger, drove home, threw the mail on her bed, and flopped on her back.

Spasms slowly gripped her spine and neck as she replayed the accident in her mind. Although she tried to remember the details clearly, the images bounced around as if she were dreaming. When her husband came home and heard her story, he decided her thinking was slow. Despite Nancy's protest that she hadn't hit her head or lost consciousness, he took her to a nearby emergency room. The doctor took X-rays of her sore neck, which turned out to be normal, and gave her pain medication, a muscle relaxant, and a foam-rubber collar for neck support. She guessed that Nancy would be better within a week.

Although the soreness in her neck and shoulders began to fade over the next two months, an almost constant dull headache persisted. Nancy traced the source of the pain by running both hands from her brows over her head and resting them on her neck. I noticed that to prevent pain when she moved, she held her neck as rigidly as she possibly could. And she slept poorly, she said, because her neck hurt when it twisted on the pillow. At night she often found herself mulling over the despair that had crept into her waking hours.

"I can't seem to do things automatically anymore," she said. "I mean, I'm incompetent, like someone on the first day of a new job."

When I asked for some examples, Nancy told me how she ordinarily set a quick pace, handling a stream of daily meetings, presentations, memos, and phone calls. She had also recently been assigned the difficult task of organizing the layoffs of nearly 50 white-collar employees. Since the accident, however, she almost always lost track of what she was doing if a colleague or phone call interrupted her. She snapped at anyone who sought her failing attention. If she did not keep notes during a conversation or meeting, she forgot key details. Yet she could not write while someone spoke and still keep up with what was being said.

"What is wrong with me?" she pleaded tearfully. "Before the accident I'd get tension headaches, but they didn't interfere with my work."

I handed Nancy a box of tissues and examined her. Her neck and shoulder girdle muscles felt tight, and pressure over several tender areas just below the back of the skull caused pain in her temples. But her strength, balance, memory, language skills, and judgment tested normal, and she was very bright and perceptive. Still, from what she had told me, she would fall apart when tasks competed for her attention. This coordination—one of the highest functions of the human brain—is orchestrated by the frontal lobes, and pain, poor sleep, and depression can overwhelm the complex mechanisms for concentrating and shifting attention. But something more seemed to be going on here.

I upped the ante in my testing to see if I could bring out the impairment. I asked Nancy to add a series of single digits two at a time, adding the second to the first, the third to the second, and so on. I gave her the series 8, 6, 9, 3, 5. She added the first two, which equaled 14, and correctly added the 9 to the preceding 6, which equaled 15. But then she stumbled by adding the 3 to 15 instead of to the preceding 9 and the 5 to the sum 18, instead of to the 3. When I corrected her, she added only the first two sums correctly and couldn't work the rest of the sequence.

Nancy's slowed responses and the dazed, dreamlike state she described following the accident reminded me of someone with a concussion from a minor head injury. In Nancy's case, I suspected the violent front and rear jolts had sheared and stretched the delicate, gelatinous tissue of her brain. The frontal lobes might even have whacked against the bony skull, creating scattered microscopic tears in some of the connections between neurons, the cells that transmit messages in the brain. When trauma like this occurs, some of the long nerve fibers that carry signals ball up and retract, and chemical messengers that enable neurons to communicate with one another get dislodged, interfering with the smooth commerce of cognitive messages.

Although the amount of tissue damage was probably slight, any injury to the brain can have dramatic consequences on thinking. I asked why she had not gone back to a doctor before seeing me.

"It was just a whiplash, I kept telling myself. I didn't want to take off a lot of time just for some headaches."

I explained that it was still worthwhile to try physical therapy for her neck and added that an antidepressant at night might help her sleep and feel less blue. I suggested that she try to limit the demands on her at work. She could hold the line on getting caught up in multiple tasks, tape-record important meetings and later make notes, and take time to rehearse what she wanted to say at meetings. I sent a note to her boss explaining her limitations and asking for his cooperation for a few months. I also arranged for a magnetic resonance imaging scan of Nancy's brain to reassure her that no unsuspected complication was interfering with her gradual recovery.

As she left, Nancy shook my hand and said, "Thanks for letting me know that I'm not going crazy."

Three weeks later the headaches were gone. Nancy moved more fluidly and she could sleep through the night. But she still felt frightened and vulnerable. "All along," she began, "I've kept up hope I'd be myself again. But it's just so grim not to be able to gracefully fit things together. It's even worse when my friends and co-workers tell me I look and sound fine. They say, 'Work harder and you'll get past it.' Sure, I'm not in a cast or paralyzed or scarred or suddenly stupid. But I'm not fine. And it hurts that people—I mean, even my husband doubts me."

If an injury can't be seen, it's easy to toss away the idea that anything's really wrong. Even doctors can slip into disbelief about the symptoms patients describe after a seemingly minor head, neck, or back injury. As long ago as the 1870s, when the first laws compensating employees for work-related injuries were passed, German and English doctors came up with the term accident neurosis to describe the condition of patients who had sustained apparently minor injuries but continued to have symptoms. And today, personal-injury lawyers and health care practitioners of every bent argue over whether some patients are malingerers out for a buck, or just worried, well-meaning people who exaggerate their symptoms.

In Nancy's case, we could not point to physical evidence of a brain injury. No patches of bleeding, swelling, or other damage had shown up on her MRI scan. Even if she had cracked her skull against the windshield, the microscopic sources of her problems might have been difficult to document. While the biological basis for Nancy's cognitive symptoms could not be explained in precise physical detail, what she said was enough for me to recognize that parts of her brain—and life—were still in disarray.

Although relieved that the pain was now gone, Nancy went on to explain what had happened the previous weekend when she tried to run a few errands. She had drawn up a shopping list and made a note to get gas and pick up clothes at the dry cleaner. But while she was driving, she couldn't decide which errand to do first. If she went to the market, her frozen foods might melt while she waited at the gas station and cleaner. On the other hand, the market would be crowded if she didn't get there by 10 a.m. She could go to the cleaner, but it was a bit out of the way, and her gas gauge read close to empty. A fill-up, though, often took a while, because her car leaked oil and that had to be checked. But then, the lines at the market were terrible on Saturdays. . . . Bewildered, she pulled over and cried. This executive with an MBA could no longer set priorities for even a simple list of errands.

"I know the stuff is in here," she said, tapping her head, "but I'm so afraid that the loose connections will never mend." I reminded her that they can and do when the damage, like hers, is limited. And I silently hoped that time would soon restore her brain's intricate electrical and chemical signaling processes to normal. The repair was overdue; most people recover within six to twelve weeks.

I tried a higher dose of the antidepressant drug, but stopped it after two weeks when it didn't seem to help. I decided to ask Nancy's husband to be more supportive. As it turned out, her boss understood her problem a lot better than her husband did. He told Nancy he had suffered a slight concussion while playing rugby in college, and for two months his concentration and memory were so poor that he barely passed his courses. So he gave Nancy what he wished his teachers had given him: He let her take on one assignment at a time, and he scheduled a weekly session with a rehabilitation therapist to help her organize her work load.

By the fourth month after the accident, Nancy told me about several mornings when her energy was high and she could concentrate on whatever was thrown at her. She zipped through the addition test that had stumped her before. By six months, the deep fear that she might never recover gave way to the pleasure of handling most of the demands she faced.

In the eighth month Nancy declared herself recovered. "I feel light and clear again," she told me. "It's as though my mind has finally pulled out of that surreal line of slow-moving traffic."

Bruce H. Dobkin, MD, FRCP, is Medical Director of the UCLA Neurologic Rehabilitation and Research Program.

CHAPTER
37

HEAVY METAL

By Daniel C. Weaver

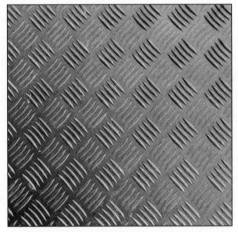

Photo 37-1

As I thumbed through the first few inches of the more than foot-thick chart, it became apparent that this was a case in which things didn't quite add up. The chart described the medical ordeal of a 35-year-old man, George Decker, a nonsmoker who had worked as a laborer in a local metal shop. He had been in perfect health until three months earlier, when he suddenly developed pneumonia in both lungs. Pneumonia can be defined as any inflammation of the lungs that causes white blood cells and cellular debris to collect in the air sacs, a condition that makes breathing difficult. In practice, most pneumonias are caused by some sort of microorganism. Yet in Mr. Decker's case, repeated cultures of the sputum he coughed up—cultures examined for bacteria, fungi, or viruses—had all come back negative.

Other causes of inflammation had been ruled out as well: As far as Mr. Decker knew, he hadn't inhaled any toxins or parasites or breathed any fluid into his lungs. His doctors eventually resorted to an open-lung biopsy to see if they could uncover the pathogen, but they found only tissue injury and repair. Over the next three months, they watched helplessly as Mr. Decker's lungs thickened, steadily undermining his ability to breathe. Eventually, after months of tests, ventilator support, failed treatments, and desperate acts, he slipped away for reasons unknown.

Now it was my job to find out why. I'm a pathologist, one of the odd birds of medicine. Although we're best known for performing autopsies (à la Quincy), we actually spend most of our time peering through microscopes at tiny snippets of tissue—called biopsies—in an attempt to understand a patient's problem. Our role is that of final arbiter: to decide if a lump is benign or malignant, if a disease is a rare infection or a weird genetic disorder. This day, my job was to piece together into a coherent diagnostic whole the story of this man's demise.

I checked the toe tag, snapped a blade into a handle, and with strong strokes cut through the skin, down to bone. I made three such cuts: one from each shoulder diagonally to what is called the xiphoid process, a bit of cartilage found at the bottom of the breastbone; and a third from there down to the pubic bone. This opened up the whole torso. I peeled back the skin and removed first the ribs and then the lungs. As I held them, cool in my hands, it was obvious that his had been a hopeless plight. The lungs, usually as light and airy as cotton candy, were as heavy and thick as a liver.

After performing a gross visual examination of all the organs, I selected small pieces of each to be processed into slides. Days later, when I studied the sections of lung under the microscope, the reason for all that weight was clear. In healthy lungs, good, oxygen-rich air is drawn down into tiny air sacs called alveoli. The alveoli in turn are wrapped in a meshwork of capillaries, so that only thin, delicate membranes separate the air from the blood; oxygen can easily and quickly get across. It is this oxygen, bound to the hemoglobin in red blood cells, that gives us the roses in our cheeks. In turn, carbon dioxide—a waste product of metabolism—travels back across the same membranes and is exhaled. But in Mr. Decker's lungs, these delicate membranes had become a dense, impenetrable thicket of debris—clot-forming proteins, inflammatory cells, and collagen—a cellular junkyard. The oxygen molecules would have had no chance to traverse this barrier and reach the blood flowing past in the capillaries. Thus, although he could draw air into his lungs, the oxygen could not get to the blood. Nor could the carbon dioxide make its way to the lungs to be exhaled. Mr. Decker had suffocated.

Still, the reason this junk had collected in his lungs remained unknown. My stains for bacteria, fungi, viruses, and parasites were all negative. In the tissues I examined, there were no telltale signs to explain why all this had happened.

Stumped, I returned to the chart. There, in notes made by a third-year medical student on the day Mr. Decker first showed up at the hospital, was my first clue. This bilingual student reported on a conversation he'd had with Mr. Decker's Spanish-speaking girlfriend, who told him that on July 3, Mr. Decker had just finished cooking when he began wheezing, coughing, and gasping for air. She'd accompanied him to the hospital, but he wasn't happy about being there. Indeed, he'd taken a swing at the nurses even though he was still breathless. The doctors treated him for an upper respiratory infection, and then, against their advice, he left. The next day he returned to the hospital, his skin tinged blue from lack of oxygen. By itself, the blue coloration didn't mean much; any bad pneumonia, severe lung infection, or major injury to lung tissue can result in the same discoloration. But that it had happened so quickly struck me as somehow important.

I needed to ask some questions. Mr. Decker's girlfriend, it turned out, was nowhere to be found. But at the top of the admission sheet, on the first page of the chart, was the name of his employer—a Mr. Wilson. I called Mr. Wilson, identifying myself as the medical examiner investigating the death of George Decker. After a long pause, he quietly agreed to answer my questions.

I began by asking exactly what it was that Mr. Decker had done in the metal shop. Mr. Wilson told me that he poured aluminum ingots. Then I simply asked, "What kind of guy was Mr. Decker?"

"Oh, he was a fellow on his way to *mucho dinero*," came the reply.

I was intrigued. "Well, how did he get *mucho dinero*?" I asked.

"Any way he could."

I paused a moment, then plunged right in. The ways Mr. Decker used—were they on the up-and-up?

"You could say no," he replied carefully.

As I listened to Mr. Wilson, my intuition took over. I had a strong hunch about what might be going on here, but I needed more information. I remembered that Mr. Decker's girlfriend said he'd been cooking just before he got sick. I asked Mr. Wilson, "Do you know what he was cooking?"

"No, not exactly," came yet another careful answer. I decided to backtrack.

"Well then, do you know how he got his money, besides by pouring aluminum ingots?"

He paused, took a deep breath, and to my surprise decided to answer me. George collected old fillings from dentists' offices and extracted the gold and silver.

"What did he do with the metal?" I continued probing. Cagily, Mr. Wilson replied that he didn't know, but he volunteered the seemingly unconnected information that in the past year alone Mr. Decker and his girlfriend had made three trips to Colombia.

I closed with one final question: Did Mr. Decker use drugs?

Again he paused, inhaled, and replied, "I personally never saw Decker use drugs."

"Thank you," I said, before hanging up. That had been an overly specific denial if ever I'd heard one. The man was a regular Henry Kissinger. It was all the confirmation I needed.

The story was beginning to unfold. The way I saw it, Mr. Decker was acquiring dental fillings, extracting the gold and silver using his vocational skills from the metal shop, and traveling to Colombia to buy drugs. But how was this connected to the pneumonia and his death?

A call to my dentist and later to a dental laboratory gave me the information I needed. They explained to me that gold fillings are actually an alloy of gold, palladium, and other metals, and that silver fillings are essentially an amalgam of silver and mercury, though tin, zinc, and copper can also be added. Gold is a heavy, impervious metal that in a pure state is soft—far too soft to withstand the gnashing of teeth. To serve as a tooth replacement, the gold is mixed with palladium; the final alloy is both tough and resistant to the acidic environment found in the mouth. The alloy is made by heating the metals in their proper proportions and then letting them cool; reheating will separate them. Gold melts at 1,945 degrees Fahrenheit, which is much lower than the melting point of palladium. So as the fillings are heated, the gold melts first and can be poured off, leaving the other metals behind.

Mr. Decker would have been fine if he had confined himself to gold fillings. But he got greedy and also went after the silver fillings, which are much more abundant. His chief job here was to separate silver from mercury. Mercury—nicknamed quicksilver—is a liquid at room temperature. When combined with other metals and cooled it stays solid, but it becomes a gas at the fairly low temperature of 674 degrees. To get the silver out of the fillings, then, Mr. Decker must have heated them until the mercury boiled off, leaving behind the silver.

In its liquid form, mercury is surprisingly nontoxic—people have ingested ounces with little effect—because it has such a high surface tension that it balls up easily, leaving very little surface area available to interact with the body. But when heated, mercury becomes an invisible, odorless toxic gas. Vaporized mercury atoms can be inhaled deep into the lungs, where they diffuse across the delicate membranes and enter the red blood cells.

Red cells contain oxidative enzymes that catalyze the linking of oxygen to hemoglobin. But when mercury gets into the bloodstream, these same enzymes oxidize it instead, yielding a highly reactive ion that destroys anything with which it comes in contact. As a consequence, mercury becomes a molecular hand grenade in which the pin has ironically been pulled by the blood itself. And as the mercury ions run rampant through the lung tissue—as they can through other tissues, including those of the brain, which would explain Mr. Decker's combativeness—they do more than just destroy it: They incite a riot of inflammation as the body desperately attempts to repair the cellular chaos. If enough mercury has been sucked into the lungs, the tissue damage and inflammation result in irreversible pneumonia and death.

And that is what I hypothesized had happened to George Decker. What I needed to do now was confirm the cause and mechanism of his death. I sent off small scraps of the lung tissue to the laboratory, which reported that though months had passed, traces of mercury were still present. So it was definitely mercury poisoning. To be sure about how the poisoning had occurred, I called the Occupational Safety and Health Administration and asked agents to test Mr. Decker's home for heavy metals. The next week they reported that beneath the floorboards adjacent to the stove they had found mercury at more than 1,000 times permissible levels. The day he got sick—July 3—George Decker had been cooking teeth in his kitchen.

When I filled out the final autopsy report, I listed Mr. Decker's cause of death as irreversible diffuse alveolar damage as a consequence of heavy metal intoxication, a long-winded way of saying his lungs failed. But as the surgeon Richard Selzer once wrote, autopsies give us the facts but not the truth. George Decker had indeed died of lung failure, but I wonder if the cause of his death wasn't far less exotic. It seems to me that he died from a combination of two of the oldest and most insidious killers of all: ignorance and avarice.

Daniel C. Weaver has thirty years of experience specializing in anatomic and clinical pathology.

CHAPTER

38

THE ARETHA FRANKLIN TEST

By Daniel C. Weaver

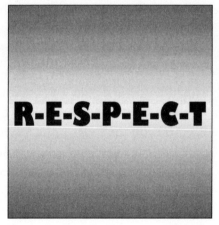

Photo 38-1

"Hey, hey. What's up, Doc?"
I glanced up from the microscope into the face of Greg
Jackson, radiologist. We were in the CT scanner room, where I

was examining tissue extracted from a tumor in a young woman's chest.

"Something's up," I replied, "but I don't know just what."

"I thought you pathologists knew it all," teased Greg.

"Well, this time I don't. I've still got scar tissue and those strange glands in the biopsy—but I can't figure out what they have to do with her lung tumor. Go ahead and do one more needle biopsy and maybe I'll find something else."

Our patient, Mrs. Henley, was a young mother with two sons, and until a week earlier, she had been perfectly healthy. Now she lay on the hard table of the CT scanner believing she had cancer, because that's what most people believe when a doctor tells them they have a tumor. But the word tumor is descriptive, not diagnostic; it is used to describe any unusual mass. When the tumor is in the lung, the cause might be cancer, pneumonia, a foreign object, or a genetic fluke. The precise nature of Mrs. Henley's tumor was what Greg and I were trying to figure out.

Mrs. Henley's nightmare had begun the previous Saturday afternoon while she was playing with her sons in the park. She had just put her younger boy on the teeter-totter when she suddenly gasped for air, fell to her knees, and grabbed her right side. Her breathing was shallow and rapid, and it hurt whether she breathed in or out. Her husband brought her in to the emergency room at a local hospital.

In a healthy person, there are only two likely reasons for sudden shortness of breath: a collapsed lung, or a foreign object blocking the flow of air. When the ER doctors tapped on the right side of Mrs. Henley's chest, they heard a drum-like echo instead of the normal dull thud. That suggested that her lung had collapsed, filling the surrounding chest cavity with air. An X-ray confirmed the suspicion. They also found a tiny bit of fluid in her right lung cavity. But they didn't find anything that would explain the collapsed lung or the extra fluid.

The ER doctors extracted the fluid with a syringe and sent it to the lab for analysis. After the removal of the fluid, Mrs. Henley's lung re-expanded. But an X-ray revealed a dense, forbidding mass in the bottom part of her right lung. To the radiologist on duty, it looked like cancer. Yet cancer alone is unlikely to cause a lung to collapse.

One of life's ironies is that the only reason we can breathe at all is because our lungs inhabit a vacuum. Imagine that the lungs are a balloon and the chest is a vacuum jar. The air pressure in the balloon is greater than the air pressure in the jar. Break the jar or puncture the balloon, and the air pressure across the balloon and the jar becomes the same. The same thing happens when the lung or the chest wall is punctured. The naturally elastic fibers of the lung collapse, just like a popped balloon. Once a lung has collapsed, the patient gasps for air.

So far, we knew two things. Something had produced a mass in Mrs. Henley's lung, and something had punctured the lung.

The next step was to look over the lab results. When Dr. Dreiser, the local pathologist, had first examined the fluid drawn from the lung, he had found a mix of strange glands and blood. He suspected that the fluid, the hole in the lung, and the mass in the chest were all caused by the same thing: adenocarcinoma, a type of glandular cancer that may have either grown in her lung or spread from some hidden site. But it would take a biopsy of the lung tumor to confirm the diagnosis. That's why Mrs. Henley was referred to our hospital, and that is what Greg and I were doing that Thursday morning in the radiology department.

We were using a CT scanner, one of modern medicine's most sophisticated instruments, to pinpoint the tumor in Mrs. Henley's chest. A CT scanner takes a series of X-rays in a rotating plane and then reassembles them to form a three-dimensional image of the body. Using the image from the CT scan to guide him, Greg inserted a thin needle through the skin directly above the tumor and drew out a few drops. I smeared those drops of blood and cells on a glass slide and stained them with two dyes.

Staining is one of cell biology's oldest techniques. One dye stains the nucleus of a cell a deep midnight blue; the other stains the rest of the cell—the cytoplasm—a brilliant sunset red. Judging from the pattern and color of the cells, the pathologist must make the final diagnosis.

Benign or malignant, good news or bad—it must seem so simple to decide. And many times for the pathologist it is. The malignant cells scream out CANCER: their nuclei are misshapen like deformed faces; their cytoplasm, filled with tissue-destroying enzymes, is swollen like a bloated belly; and their growth is murderously uncontrolled. But sometimes cancerous cells are sneaky little devils, artfully dressed like wolves in sheep's clothing, stealthily insinuating themselves around healthy cells until they can silently throttle them. The pathologist's task is to decide whether the odd-looking cells are good guys in a bad mood or charming, handsome mass murderers like Ted Bundy.

Dreiser suspected cancer, but I wasn't so sure. There are many signs of cancer, none of them definitive on their own. A cell with a large nucleus filled with dark, distorted DNA is one sign of a malignant cell. The rapid growth and spread of these cells to other organs is another. But the single most helpful sign in deciding whether cells are benign or malignant is what I call the Aretha

Franklin sign: R-E-S-P-E-C-T. If the odd cells—no matter how tortured or ugly or proliferative—show respect for themselves and respect for their neighbors, they are overwhelmingly likely to be benign.

To my eye, Mrs. Henley's unusual-looking cells showed this respect. They were neatly arranged in little groups that didn't disrupt the functioning of other cells. Their nuclei didn't look as dark and densely packed as the nuclei of cancerous cells, which often have twice the normal amount of DNA. Moreover, these cells didn't have the shoved-around look of misshapen nuclei and squashed cytoplasm that often betrays the presence of cancer. These cells might be misbehaving, but I wasn't so sure they were cancerous. They just seemed lost. But what were they doing in the lung? Why did they punch a hole in it? And why did they make a mass like a cancer?

Another ten minutes of thought got me no closer to an answer. "Greg, the last pass through the lung was it. You certainly hit it. I've just got to think what it means."

I considered the possibilities: Cancer? Infection? A genetic disorder? Cancer, whether it arises in the lungs or arrives from elsewhere, is certainly the most common cause of lung tumors—but not in 27-year-old women. Besides, the cells I saw here just didn't look like cancer. They were a bit ugly and distorted, but they passed the Aretha Franklin test. Yet I couldn't be certain. Perhaps this was an extraordinary kind of cancer that violated this most important rule of biology. Or perhaps this was a hamartoma—a rare genetic aberration in which the normal proportion of benign lung cells is out of whack. But that would require the presence of two or more kinds of cells, and I saw only one. And it would not explain the presence of blood in the fluid. Was this an infection? If so, why did she have no history of pneumonia or even a fever? I decided to sleep on it.

In the morning, I began again with the slides of Mrs. Henley's lung tumor. I placed the slide of cells under the microscope and scanned across the cellular horizon. Enmeshed in a sea of blood were deep blue nuclei arranged in circles like wagon trains on a dusty red desert. I switched to a higher magnification to get a closer look. The nuclei were large and evenly blue, arranged in discrete ovals and circles. In the cytoplasm were tiny bubbles—a sign of secretions from the mysterious glands.

But just knowing there were glands in Mrs. Henley's lung tissue didn't help me much. Glands are very common in nearly every organ. They coat the gullet, lungs, and womb, and they make sweat, milk, and tears. The cells that make up glands are easy to spot because they cluster in rings, forming a hole to let out their secretions. The inner surface of the lungs normally contains glands that secrete fluids to prevent the lungs from drying out. But one place that glands absolutely don't belong is on the outer surface of the lungs, where there is no place to discharge their secretions. That's where Mrs. Henley's funny-looking glands were. I knew they didn't belong there, but that was all I could say for sure. Who were these guys? What were they doing? What were they trying to secrete?

I flipped back to the lower magnification, then switched once more to the higher magnification and peered again at these midnight blue cells. This time I saw something I hadn't noticed before. Just to the side of the wagon trains of blue cells were small, narrow, spindle-shaped companions stained a very pale blue. It suddenly dawned on me who these small companions were. They were stromal cells, a kind of cell that supports many organs.

The presence of stromal cells beside the puzzling glands could mean only one thing. This wasn't cancer. This was endometriosis.

Endometriosis is a strange and, to the pathologist, wondrous disorder. The endometrium is a thin coating of glands and stromal cells that lines the uterus. Occasionally—and for unknown reasons—these benign cells migrate from the lining of the uterus to other parts of the body. Usually they spread across the surface of the ovaries or fallopian tubes. But occasionally they can spread to the belly button, the skin, or in rare cases, to the surface of the lung. No matter where they spread, no matter how far from the endometrium, these cells will often still respond to a woman's hormonal cycle.

When a woman's hormones signal the start of the menstrual cycle, the growth of the endometrial cells—estranged or not—is disrupted, and the endometrial lining decays. When that sloughing begins, it ruptures the tiny blood vessels that support the endometrial lining, which starts the menstrual flow. When endometrial tissue is growing outside the uterus, however, this cellular sloughing can damage the surrounding tissue. If the endometrial tissue is growing on the fallopian tubes, it can cause infertility. In Mrs. Henley's case, the endometrial growth damaged the surface of the lung, causing the bleeding we had detected. And if there is enough abnormal growth, it may form scar tissue or even punch a hole in the thin, lacy surface of the lung. That kind of growth would also explain Mrs. Henley's collapsed lung and lung tumor.

When I called Greg to fill him in, he was surprised and pleased that we had at last found the source of the mysterious glands. Later in the day I went upstairs to Mrs. Henley's floor and read over her chart. When I stopped by her room, I found her lying in bed on her left side, a position that probably relieved some of the pain in her right lung.

"Hello, I'm Dr. Weaver, one of the specialists here," I began. "Would you mind if I ask you a few questions?"

"Go ahead. I'm feeling much better now that the doctors told me what it really is."

"From what I read on your chart, I see that you've had shortness of breath many times with your periods. Did your doctor ever try to figure out what was going on?"

"No, we just thought I had bad cramps."

"Well, did the shortness of breath ever go away for several months in a row?"

"Sure," she replied, "when I was pregnant with each of my boys."

Just as the stromal cells had gone undetected, sometimes the truth lies before us, just too obvious to see.

Later Mrs. Henley's gynecologist explained to her the ways to treat endometriosis. Basically, there are just two methods, and neither works very well. One treatment uses hormones to alter the signals the endometrium receives, essentially creating a state of false pregnancy. The other uses lasers to burn away the excess endometrial growth. Mrs. Henley chose the hormonal treatment, and for a few months at least she has had no recurrence. But endometriosis is rarely eliminated for good. Symptoms can return even if the most common sites of growth—the ovaries and uterus—are completely excised. Until there is a cure for endometriosis, the best that Mrs. Henley can hope to achieve is an uneasy truce with her disorder.

Daniel C. Weaver has thirty years of experience specializing in anatomic and clinical pathology.

CHAPTER

39

THE POULTICE OF TIME

By Daniel C. Weaver

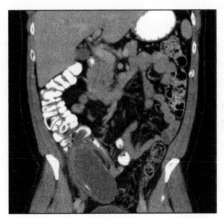

Photo 39-1

"What did you find?" I asked Jeff as he walked into the doctors' lounge.

"Not much. Just looked like guts to me," Jeff replied. "I thought cancer or a ruptured appendix might explain the pain," he added, "but as far as I could tell there was nothing in that boy's belly but normal bowel. Maybe you'll find something in the bone marrow—all I know for sure is that he is sicker than a dog that's been wormed."

Our patient, J. J. Walker, had recently been hospitalized because of excruciating abdominal pain. Jeff had just completed a laparotomy—a surgical exploration of the abdomen. He had made an incision from Mr. Walker's navel to his pubis, then looked at the organs closely, feeling for any abnormalities in the bowels, liver, stomach, and spleen. But he had come up empty-handed. There was nothing apparent to the naked eye or the soft touch of a gloved hand to explain why Mr. Walker was in such pain. As a pathologist, I would have the job of hunting for clues in the bone marrow.

Jeff and I work at a hospital in Columbus, Ohio, but Mr. Walker's story had begun over 200 miles away in a small town tucked away in the hollows of the foothills of the Appalachian Mountains. He had woken up three days earlier, on November 11, with a pain deep in his belly. It was a Sunday morning. For the next four hours he had remained at the commode, vomiting. Finally he asked his wife to take him to a nearby hospital in Shepherd, Ohio.

Providence Hospital is a small, old facility that serves one of the state's most impoverished counties. The land there is tough and poor, and the people reflect their geography. They are craggy, stoic, and nearly unbreakable. I'm asked to visit the hospital from time to time, and the biggest tumors I've seen—some the size of a rat—come out of those hollows. When a man from a hollow yelps, I know he's not crying wolf.

When Mr. Walker arrived in the emergency room, the laboratory technicians drew blood for standard tests and took a urine sample for a routine drug screen. The most common cause of intense abdominal pain in a 24-year-old man is acute appendicitis, and that was the working diagnosis until the test results came back.

Mr. Walker's urine test was normal, showing no trace of drug use or infection. But his blood count was extremely low for all three kinds of blood cells: the red cells that carry oxygen, the white cells that fight infection, and the platelets that help blood clot. J. J. Walker had bad blood, but no one knew why. My colleague Ed Bains, a blood specialist, was called down to Shepherd from the hospital in Columbus where we work.

On Monday afternoon, Ed examined Mr. Walker for the first time. Tall, angular, and a bit abrupt, Ed is like many hematologist-oncologists I have known who every day have to deliver to perfectly lovely people the perfectly awful news of blood disorders or cancer.

Mr. Walker's belly was as taut as a drum—often a sign that the bowel is about to burst. Ed couldn't tell what was going wrong, but he had a hunch. Belly pain and bad blood are common signs of lymphoma, a cancer of the white blood cells. The primary targets in patients with lymphoma are the lymph nodes—bits of tissue scattered about the body where white blood cells and other immune cells exchange the signals that promote healthy immune function. Attacks on the numerous lymph nodes that line the bowel could have been the source of Mr. Walker's belly pain. In addition, renegade white blood cells could have been taking over Mr. Walker's bone marrow, disturbing the normal production of blood cells. The only way to know for sure would be to look for abnormalities in Mr. Walker's bowel and bone marrow.

Ed explained the need for exploratory surgery to Mr. Walker and his wife and recommended that Mr. Walker be transferred to our hospital in Columbus. A CT scanner there could detect any enlarged lymph nodes. After a four-hour ambulance ride through the hills and onto the flats of central Ohio, Mr. Walker arrived at our hospital on Monday evening. The next day's efforts were dead ends. Nothing showed up on the CT scan, and Jeff found nothing wrong in Mr. Walker's belly. Ed then extracted a bit of Mr. Walker's bone marrow for me to examine.

On Wednesday morning I slid the sample under the microscope and twisted the knob to bring the blood cells into focus. Buried so deep within us, the marrow is the very soul of the blood, and what cruel and extraordinary tales it can tell. But Mr. Walker's marrow was strangely silent. His red blood cells were a bit swollen, or megaloblastic, and stippled with tiny clumps of hemoglobin and iron. Those scattered clumps, called basophilic stippling, are a very general sign that the red blood cells aren't making hemoglobin properly. It occurs in disorders as diverse as anemia, malaria, and vitamin deficiencies.

But I saw nothing that could explain why Mr. Walker's bone marrow wasn't releasing normal amounts of blood cells. The proportion of red blood cells, white blood cells, and cells that become platelets was just about right. There was no sign of murderously multiplying cancer cells. So far I had turned up nothing in Mr. Walker's bone marrow to link the blood and the belly.

I called Ed. "Close, but no cigar. Just some fat red blood cells and some stippling. What do you think?"

"Well, I'll check for a vitamin deficiency, but I don't think it means much." On Mr. Walker's fifth day in the hospital, his condition took a turn for the worse. His feet began to tingle. By the next Wednesday he couldn't move his toes, and by the following Friday his lower legs were nearly paralyzed. Now we had three conditions—abdominal pain, failing blood, and nerve damage—

and no causes. After nearly two weeks of work, Ed and I were going nowhere. Mr. Walker was receiving fluids and other supportive care, but he was slipping from our grasp. In desperation I went up to Mr. Walker's ward and carefully reviewed his chart.

Until he was admitted to the hospital, J. J. Walker had been in perfect health. He came in for belly pain with no visible cause. His blood cell counts were low, but his bone marrow was normal. Now, two weeks after he was admitted, his muscles and nerves were beginning to fail.

Clearly something was knocking out Mr. Walker's gut, blood, and nerves that we couldn't see with our eyes or a microscope. It had to be something even smaller than a single cell. Most likely it was a molecule—perhaps some kind of poison.

Mr. Walker's drug test had been negative, but it had screened only for the most commonly abused drugs. There are thousands upon thousands of poisons. It could be a heavy metal. It could be snake venom. It could be an overdose of a prescription drug or an over-the-counter medication. It could be toxic fumes from a manufacturing plant. Each poison requires a specific test to detect it. Unless I had a hunch, I would be ordering tests in the dark. Then, as I was closing the chart, I noticed Mr. Walker's occupation: plumber. Could this be lead poisoning? If Mr. Walker had welded pipes with lead solder, he might have accidentally inhaled lead as it vaporized.

I called Ed. "What about lead poisoning?" I asked. "That would explain the abdominal pain, the problems in the blood, and even the nerve damage."

"Good idea, but lead would cause paralysis without tingling. It only affects the nerves that supply muscle, not the sensory nerves."

"I know, but it's still a possibility."

"Okay. I'll order a screen for heavy metals."

That screen would test for metals with high atomic mass, such as lead, mercury, and platinum. A device called an atomic absorption spectrometer detects the presence of heavy metals in a patient's urine sample. Each metal absorbs at its own particular wavelength—254 nanometers for mercury, 283 for lead, and so on. By bombarding the sample with radiation and observing which wavelengths were being absorbed, we could tell whether a heavy metal was poisoning Mr. Walker. Two days later I reviewed the results. They were positive, but not for what I thought. What was killing Mr. Walker wasn't lead but something far more poisonous. It was arsenic, a molecule so reactive that it can bind to nearly every cell in the body, with protean and devastating effects.

In its most common form, arsenic is nearly tasteless, and once ingested, it quickly produces intense abdominal pain. First the gut absorbs the poison. Then the arsenic enters the bloodstream and is carried from head to toe and to every organ in between. If enough poison is ingested, arsenic kills instantly. If not, the poisoning gradually disrupts the body's normal functions. Blood cell production in the bone marrow will falter, and two to three weeks after the initial poisoning, the tingling and paralysis of the hands and feet begin.

I called Ed with the news.

"We finally nailed it," he exclaimed. "We've finally found something to unite what's happening in Mr. Walker's gut, blood, and nerves."

"Now we've got to find out how it happened."

This time Ed had a few hunches. Mr. Walker might have been exposed to arsenic accidentally, possibly at work. He might even have attempted suicide. Or he might have been intentionally poisoned.

While Ed headed off to question Mr. Walker, I returned to the lab and began my own investigation. Arsenic kills by attaching to sulfhydryl groups, highly reactive molecules that are required for the function of many energy-producing enzymes. Because hair and nails are rich in sulfhydryl groups and grow at known rates, I would be able to tell when Mr. Walker was poisoned by locating exactly where arsenic showed up on a shaft of his hair.

When I asked Ed to get a lock of Mr. Walker's hair, he learned that Mr. Walker's wife had recently cut her husband's hair and nails very short. I then asked Ed to get a sample of what was left and to mark clearly which end had been closest to the head.

Ed sent me an inch-long sample, bound with a red rubber band at one end. Hair grows about .37 millimeters a day, so the sample would provide a record of 60 days' growth. I divided the shaft into portions 3 millimeters long, each portion reflecting about one week's growth. Then I began the tests for arsenic.

I had a feeling some things in this case didn't add up.

When J. J. Walker arrived at the ER in Shepherd, his blood cell count was already extremely low. If the poisoning was recent, that shouldn't have happened for another day or two. What's more, nerve damage showed up within 5 days, not the usual 14 to 21 days.

Two days later, on November 23, my analysis was complete. J. J. Walker had had a whopping dose of arsenic about two weeks earlier. That would correspond with his admission to the hospital on November 11. A week before that, he had had a little dose of arsenic. And three weeks earlier, sometime in the last week of October, Mr. Walker had had another big dose. I called Ed and told him what I'd found.

When Ed explained the results to Mr. Walker, he learned that Mr. Walker had had a bout of flu around Halloween—about three weeks earlier.

Ed asked investigators from the Occupational Safety and Health Administration to inspect Mr. Walker's home and workplaces, but no trace of arsenic was found. Ed even had Mr. Walker evaluated by a psychiatrist, who informed us that he wasn't suicidal. Then the Bureau of Criminal Investigation set to work on the case. They began by closely questioning Mr. Walker's wife. But no arsenic was ever found and no admissions were made.

During the next two months, Mr. Walker got worse, despite continuous treatment with a drug that binds up arsenic. The paralysis crept up his legs toward his chest until he needed a respirator to breathe. Then slowly, a cell at a time it seemed, the nerves began to fire again and the paralysis receded like a poisonous tide.

Over the course of his hospitalization, Mr. Walker learned that his wife was having an affair with his best friend. The Walkers divorced, and she moved in with the friend. Finally, months after he was first admitted, he hobbled out of the hospital and headed home alone, a cane in either hand.

J. J. Walker still lives in Shepherd, just about 100 yards from the Ohio River. Occasionally his mother lays a warm mustard poultice across his legs, hoping to draw out the poison. On a good day he says he can make it down to the river and back in about an hour. With time the nerves in his legs are recovering, but I doubt they will ever be the same. And I suspect that even the poultice of time cannot erase the scars on J. J. Walker's heart.

Daniel C. Weaver has thirty years of experience specializing in anatomic and clinical pathology.

CHAPTER

40

THE SECRET IN THE MARROW

By Daniel C. Weaver

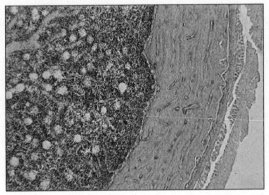

Photo 40-1

As I rode the hospital elevator up to Mrs. Fortner's room, I reviewed the case in my mind. This 42-year-old woman had gone to a clinic, complaining that she was tired and weak. A doctor there had taken blood and noted a very low red blood cell count, as well as a slightly elevated white cell count.

"Iron-deficiency anemia," he told his patient. "You have iron-poor blood." The white count he chalked up to a slight infection. He sent her over to our hospital for a more thorough blood workup. But when Julia Jones, our hematologist, looked under a microscope, she focused on the white cells. She saw oval nuclei and bluish cytoplasm.

They looked peculiar, she thought. Indeed, they all looked like plasma cells, specialized antibody-making cells not normally found in the blood. And there were lots of them: It looked like they were growing unchecked, out of control, like plasma-cell leukemia.

That's when Julia called me. I'm a pathologist, a sort of doctor's doctor—a detective, even, armed with a high-powered microscope. Because we diagnose but do not treat, pathologists have the luxury to hunt down rare, bizarre disorders—what are often referred to as medical zebras. Indeed, we have an affinity for the exotic. And this certainly fit the bill: Not only is plasma-cell leukemia a very rare disease, it's mainly a disease of the elderly.

I knocked on the door and, without waiting for a reply, walked in. A pale woman with a slight anxious tremor in her hand was lying in bed.

"Hello, Mrs. Fortner, I'm Dr. Weaver," I introduced myself. "Dr. Jones asked me to come and see you. How are you doing?"

"Okay, I guess," she replied. "I'm just so tired. But Dr. Jones did say you'd be coming by this morning."

"Yes. Well, she asked me to take a sample of your bone marrow—a biopsy, it's called—so we can try to figure out why you're so tired."

"Will it hurt—the biopsy?" she asked.

"Yes, somewhat," I answered truthfully. "The pain will be sharp but short and will be gone when I am."

The technician brought in a tray with anesthetic and some needles, and I explained the procedure to Mrs. Fortner. "The bone marrow is the site where the blood cells are made," I said. "By analyzing the bone marrow, we can see if there is anything wrong with the way your blood is fanned. To obtain a sample of the marrow, I will first numb the skin over your right hip and then insert a needle through the skin and into the center of the bone—the marrow."

To biopsy bone marrow is to drill for oil. A large-bore needle (something the size a veterinarian might use to anesthetize a horse) is inserted through the skin to the bone. When it hits bone, the doctor begins to rotate and grind the needle, to push its thick tip through the stony outer cortex. Once it has pierced the bone and reached the marrow cavity, the needle's sharp center stylet is removed, and the fluid and cells that compose the marrow are drawn through the outer shaft of the needle. Sometimes the fluid gushes out, sometimes it oozes, and sometimes it has to be sucked out by pulling back on a syringe.

I asked Mrs. Fortner to roll onto her side. I placed my hand on her hip to locate its highest, broadest point. Then I numbed the skin with an anesthetic and pushed the needle in until it butted against the bone. "It will hurt now," I warned. I firmly held the base of the assembled needle, then twisted and pushed it into the marrow cavity. Mrs. Fortner flinched but otherwise held steady. I removed the center stylet and waited for the thick, dark red marrow to ooze out into the needle hub. Normally it begins within a few seconds. But nothing came from Mrs. Former's marrow. So I attached a syringe to the needle hub and tried to aspirate the marrow. Nothing. I repositioned the needle and tried again. Still nothing.

What was going on here? I wouldn't be able to tell until I could look at the marrow. I was sure I was there—I could feel the needle give way as it passed through the cortex. So I decided to do what oil geologists sometimes do: cut a cylindrical core of material, remove it, and take it back to the laboratory.

I removed the syringe from the hub of the needle and put in its place a core cutting tool, which I slowly rotated and twisted, back and forth, until I had removed a chunk of marrow eight-tenths of an inch across. Mrs. Fortner never moved. When I was finished, I thanked her for her patience and returned to the lab to see if I could find out what strange disorder lay locked within her bones.

The bone marrow is the cellular womb of the blood. It's where the red cells (which carry oxygen), the platelets (which help blood clot), and the white cells (which help defend against bacteria and other foreign agents) are born, nurtured, and mature before being released into the bloodstream. During development, these three components grow in small, separate groupings called colonies that are supported by a delicate network of fibers known as reticulin. I needed to be able to recognize and locate these different components, so I stained the marrow with red and blue dyes. Normally the red cells stain red, the platelets stain a kind of deep blue gray, and the white cells remain basically white with a dark nucleus.

But when I looked through the microscope at Mrs. Fortner's marrow, I saw none of this. I adjusted the scope to its lowest power and looked down over the entire slide, like a bird soaring high in the sky to see a whole field below. All I could see were white cells—immature-looking white cells—spread out across the cellular landscape.

Next I adjusted the scope to its highest power, magnifying the field 1,000 times, swooping down to peer into these primeval cells. Although they had the oval nucleus Dr. Jones had described, they didn't have the characteristic clumping of genetic material found in plasma cells. They didn't even have the small cytoplasmic granules common to most white cells. These cells looked like no normal cell I knew. They weren't even like the abnormal cells I knew. They weren't piled up on one another like most tumor cells. Instead, they were remarkably evenly spaced: they looked like soldiers linked arm in arm, marching to the horizon. And as they went, they were pushing aside the normal members of the marrow community.

Who were these guys? Clearly they were traitorous desperados, despite their white hats. But where did they come from? And why hadn't any of them come out when I tried to aspirate the marrow?

I took a deep breath and decided to begin at the beginning, with the original slide of Mrs. Fortner's blood, the one Julia had looked at. I saw just what Julia had seen—a low red cell count and an increased number of white cells with oval, eccentric nuclei. Then I switched the microscope to the highest power and adjusted the light. And there it was. At the edges of the cells, at their cytoplasmic extremes, were tiny but clearly visible hair-like projections—tentacles. Plasma cells don't have tentacles. No, this was something even rarer, even more exotic. This looked like a case of hairy-cell leukemia.

What wonders a single drop of blood can reveal—malaria, leukemia, pernicious anemia, exotic fevers like Royal (which is found only in the valleys of the high Andes), and even hairy-cell leukemia, a most strange and wondrous disorder, first described just 36 years ago. As its name suggests, hairy-cell leukemia is a proliferation of a peculiar type of white cell—the hairy cell—whose tiny cytoplasm projections look like hairs under the microscope. Of course, they aren't really hairs—they're far too small—but they give these cells their singular and ominous look.

I was pretty sure about my diagnosis. But in pathology, pretty sure isn't good enough. The wrong diagnosis can lead to the wrong therapy or even death. So I ordered more tests. A test for iron showed that Mrs. Fortner's clinic doctor had been at least partly right. She did have an iron deficiency, probably from menstrual bleeding. It just wasn't the cause of her weakness.

It was when I specifically stained the reticulum—the fibers in the marrow—that I confirmed my diagnosis and finally understood why I'd had such trouble aspirating the marrow. The hairy cells were separated one from the other by precisely the length of their tentacles, and the tentacles themselves were wrapped around one another and around the reticulin fibers in a tangled mass. Like a Gordian knot, the hairy cells were literally linked arm in arm. There was no way to separate them from one another, no way to draw this mass up through the shaft of a needle.

That afternoon I called Julia to let her know what I had found. "This is an oddball case," I said, "although I'm not sure it's so much a zebra as it is an okapi."

"What? An okapi?" Julia sounded bemused.

"Yes, an okapi. One of the last great hoofed animals described by zoologists this century. It looks like a cross between a giraffe and a zebra."

"Get to the point, Weaver," Julia demanded.

"It's hairy-cell leukemia."

"Really?" she exclaimed. "That's great."

Now, doctors don't usually get excited when they hear their patient has a rare, dangerous disease. Until recently, many patients with hairy-cell leukemia died as the hairy cells crowded out the normal white cells so that the patients couldn't fight off even the simplest of infections. But thanks to a miracle of molecular biology, hairy-cell leukemia has become quite curable.

In 1972, Eloise Giblet, a Seattle hematologist and geneticist, was asked to test the blood of a child with severe combined immunodeficiency—another zebra—for a series of enzymes found in the blood cells. Dr. Giblett found that the child's blood lacked adenosine deaminase, an enzyme that helps convert adenosine, a component of DNA, into a harmless metabolite when DNA is being broken down. In this rare immune deficiency, adenosine and other metabolites accumulate in the white cells and prevent them from making more DNA, eventually resulting in their death.

Children with this immune deficiency are extremely prone to infection. Indeed, for them to survive, some have been placed in complete isolation: recall David, the boy who lived in a plastic bubble. Although David eventually succumbed to his disorder, what we learned from him and children like him is what I was counting on to help Mrs. Fortner live. It's one of the ironies of medicine that out of such dark aberrations of nature comes light.

Shortly after the discovery that white cells are exquisitely sensitive to the toxic metabolites of DNA, researchers began investigating whether they could use this information to treat proliferative dissuaders of abnormal white cells—in other words, leukemias. The idea behind the research was a simple one: to make a drug that would act like adenosine but that would kill only the bad, leukemic cells and spare the good guys.

In 1986, two years after David died, the Scripps Clinic in LaJolla, California, began treating hairy-cell leukemia with a structural mimic of adenosine called 2-chlorodeoxyadenosine. In 1990, the researchers reported that patients treated with this new drug for just one week were in complete long-term remission. For all intents and purposes, they were cured.

The week after Mrs. Fortner's diagnosis, I ran across Julia in the hallway. She seemed depressed, and for good reason. Mrs. Fortner was not a wealthy woman; her only insurance was Indiana's Medicaid program. The Medicaid officer had refused to authorize the use of the new drug because it had yet to be approved by the Food and Drug Administration. He would, however, pay for long-term conventional chemotherapy—a treatment that would only postpone Mrs. Former's demise, and at enormous expense. Despite Julia's pleas, the bureaucrats had remained immobile, and Mrs. Fortner had remained untreated.

I thought about calling Medicaid myself, but then thought better of it. I have learned over the years that bureaucrats are prisoners of rules, regulations, and lawyers; they are not in a position to evaluate new therapies. Sometimes I wonder if they realize that the enemy out there is disease.

But Julia wasn't giving up. She kept looking for an alternative source of funds. Later that week, she found it. The hospital administrator agreed to have the hospital itself absorb the cost.

Three months after her one-week treatment with 2-chlorodeoxyadenosine, I saw Mrs. Former in the hospital outpatient clinic. The tremor was gone and her cheeks were rosy. She was there so I could take another biopsy of her marrow, to make sure the therapy had worked.

"Hello, Mrs. Fortner," I said. "I'm glad to see you back."

"Oh, Dr. Weaver, I heard that you were the one who found out what was wrong with me," she replied. "I guess I owe you a thank-you."

"Well, I don't know about that, Mrs. Fortner," I said. "I was just doing my job." I felt uncomfortable and finally said, "Why don't you just get ready, and I'll complete my final biopsy." Again I placed my hand on her hip to locate its highest, broadest point, numbed the skin, and proceeded. The marrow gushed out easily.

When I had finished, however, and was on my way back to the laboratory, I thought to myself, I wish I had been a little quicker on my feet. Yes, there are some people Mrs. Fortner might want to thank, and she might want to begin with the Davids of this world.

The following day I placed the slide of Mrs. Former's bone marrow under my microscope and focused. The hairy white traitors that had once filled her bones had vanished. In their place, in all their complexity and diversity, were islands of reds, whites, and blues—a normal marrow. On February 26, 1993, the FDA approved 2-chiorodeoxyadenosine for the treatment of hairy-cell leukemia.

Daniel C. Weaver has thirty years of experience specializing in anatomic and clinical pathology.

Appendix

This appendix includes the title of each chapter and the original publication date of the articles.

Attacked from Within, May 21, 2007
Why is Grandpa Falling?, August 1, 2006
The Boy Who Stopped Talking, April 2, 2006
Why is Her Vision So Hazy?, August 1, 2006
Instant Paralysis with an Instant Cure, November 28, 2007
Why Does Her Belly Hurt?, March 10, 2006
A Sleepy Secret, December 11, 2010
What is Fanning His Temper?, March 14, 2013
Why is She Getting Thinner?, May 29, 2006
A Stress Caser or Serious Disease?, September 17, 2011
A 20-Pound, Bony Tumor That Nearly Suffocated a Man From the Inside, December 6, 2011
Far From Okay, August 1, 2006
Save the Linebacker, February 1, 2013
We Can Take His Heart Out, Remove the Tumor, and Put it Back In, May 9, 2012
An Unwelcoming Ringing, June 10, 2010
Misdiagnosing ADHD, August 22, 2007
A Swollen Area Grows Larger and Larger, June 5, 2005
High Head Pressure, January 31, 2007
A leg of Legendary Size, May 30, 2012
The Sneaky Pain That Fooled 6 Experts, August 27, 2009
One Cure for Vertigo: Playing Pinball Inside Your Head, September 10, 2008

Cruising into Trouble, August 1, 2006

The Woman Who Needed to Be Upside-Down, August 27, 2012

The Patient's Symptoms Resembled a Back Ache, but Their Cause Might Prove Far More Deadly, January 1, 2001

Why Can't This Woman Breathe?, June 27, 2004

The Disease That Shows Us How We Are What We Eat, June 27, 2004

The Blood Pressure Mystery, April 16, 2008

Mary Grove was Suddenly Shedding Skin in Large Red Patches. The Loss Was a Threat to Her Life, February 1, 1999

Benign but Irritating Skin Eruptions Signal Much More Serious Internal Troubles, November 22, 2005

A Song from *Shrek* Helps a 5-Year-Old Boy Recover from Difficult Surgery, August 6, 2005

Present Tense, August 1, 1992

Mechanic of the Mind, August 1990

The Absentminded Professor, October 1, 1992

Fighting With Phantoms, March 1, 1992

Netting the Butterfly, September 1, 1993

An Insult to the Brain, February 1, 1994

Heavy Metal, April 1, 1993

The Aretha Franklin Test, March 2, 1995

The Poultice of Time, June 1, 1995

The Secret in the Marrow, 1994